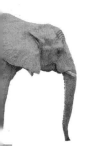

Mnemonics
for Medical
Undergraduates

Dr Shahed Yousaf
BSc(Hons) University of Wolverhampton
MB ChB Leicester-Warwick Medical Schools

Dr Mubeen A. Chaudhry
BSc(Hons) Kings College London,
University of London
MB ChB Leicester-Warwick Medical Schools

PasTest

D1144114

© 2006 PASTEST LTD
Egerton Court
Parkgate Estate
Knutsford
Cheshire
WA16 8DX

Telephone: 01565 752000

First Published 2006

ISBN: 1 904627 88 9
ISBN: 978 1904 627 883

A catalogue record for this book is available from the British Library.

Text prepared by Type Study, Scarborough, North Yorkshire

Printed and bound in the UK by MPG Books Ltd., Bodmin, Cornwall

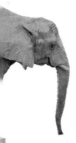

Mnemonic

1753, from the Greek *mnemonikos* 'of or pertaining to memory', from *mnemon* (gen. *mnemonos*) 'remembering, mindful', from *mnasthai* 'remember'.

Mnemosyne, lit. 'memory, remembrance', was a Titaness, mother of the Muses.

Shahed Yousaf

I would like to thank Mohammad Yousaf, Bilqees Begum and Shazadi Yousaf, who assisted in the task of assembling this book.

Mubeen Chaudhry

I would like to thank my family, in particular my mother, for encouraging me to complete this project.

and

To the countless medical students who take time to devise mnemonics in order to disseminate knowledge and make studying fun. We would like to thank the contributors to this and future editions.

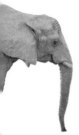

Contents

Introduction

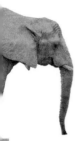

This book is written by medical students for medical students. As final-year medical students we both realised that we would need mnemonics in order to succeed in our examinations. Mnemonics allow complex information to be condensed into a few words and essentially make your memory more efficient. There is no substitute for hard work and wider reading but this is of little use if you cannot locate your facts or get information muddled up. Mnemonics allow you to secure information in your head with the aid of word play or visual associations. If a good depth of knowledge is the cake then mnemonics are the icing.

The mnemonics in this book have been created or collated by us and we have found them to be invaluable in our studies. There are many sources of mnemonics out there but it can be time-consuming to go through many phrases from different sources for the same condition. In this book we have incorporated the mnemonics that we have personally tested and found to be the most memorable. The best mnemonics are those that are most relevant and therefore it is beneficial to try and personalise them. A mnemonic should not have to try too hard or you will need a mnemonic to remember it!

The book is divided logically into medical systems such as the cardiovascular system, the gastrointestinal system, the respiratory system, etc. Each system begins with some histology and than salient anatomy, if relevant. This is followed by the clinical conditions relating to that system. All care has been taken to include mnemonics on high-yield topics. The entries reflect our opinions on what is relevant.

We actively encourage medical students and interested parties to contact us with new mnemonics or improvements to the ones

featured here (email mnemonicsformedicalundergraduates@pastest.
co.uk). We hope you enjoy this book and find it to be a worthwhile
addition to your medical library.

Shahed Yousaf

Mubeen Chaudhry

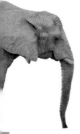

Abbreviations

ABPA	Allergic bronchopulmonary aspergillosis
ACE	Angiotensin-converting enzyme
ACTH	Adrenocorticotrophic hormone
AD	Alzheimer's disease
ADH	Antidiuretic hormone
AF	Atrial fibrillation
ANA	Anti-nuclear antibody
APD	Automated peritoneal dialysis
APH	Ante-partum haemorrhage
APKD	Adult polycystic kidney disease
ARDS	Acute respiratory distress syndrome
ARF	Acute renal failure
ASD	Atrial septal defect
AST	Aspartate aminotransferase
ATN	Acute tubular necrosis
BP	Blood pressure
BV	Bacterial vaginosis
CABG	Coronary artery bypass graft
CAPD	Continuous ambulatory peritoneal dialysis
CBG	Corticosteroid-binding globulin
CHF	Congestive heart failure
CIN	Cervical intraepithelial neoplasia
CML	Chronic myelogenous leukaemia
CMV	Cytomegalovirus
CNS	Central nervous system
COPD	Chronic obstructive pulmonary disease
CPPD	Calcium pyrophosphate dihydrate
CPR	Cardiopulmonary resuscitation
CRH	Corticotrophin-releasing hormone
CSF	Cerebro-spinal fluid
CT	Computed tomography
CTG	Cardiotocography

CVA	Cerebrovascular accident
CXR	Chest X-ray
DG	Diacylglycerol
DHEA	Dehydroepiandrosterone
DI	Diabetes insipidus
DIC	Disseminated intravascular coagulation
DIP	Distal interphalangeal
DKA	Diabetic ketoacidosis
DM	Diabetes mellitus
DVT	Deep vein thrombosis
EBV	Epstein–Barr virus
EMD	Electromechanical dissociation
EPO	Erythropoietin
ERCP	Endoscopic retrograde cholangiopancreatography
ESR	Erythrocyte sedimentation rate
ESRF	End-stage renal failure
FBC	Full blood count
FSH	Follicle-stimulating hormone
GH	Growth hormone
GHRH	GH-releasing hormone
GIFT	Gamete intrafallopian transfer
GN	Glomerulonephritis
GnRH	Gonadotropin-releasing hormone
GORD	Gastroesophageal reflux disease
GTN	Glyceryl trinitrate
HELLP	Haemolysis, elevated liver enzymes, low platelets
HIV	Human immunodeficiency virus
HMSN	Hereditary motor sensory neuropathy
HPA	Hypothalamic–pituitary–adrenal
HPOA	Hypertrophic pulmonary osteoarthropathy
HPV	Human papilloma virus
HRT	Hormone replacement therapy
HSP	Henoch–Schonlein purpura
HSV	Herpes simplex virus
HTN	Hypertension
HUS	Haemolytic–uraemic syndrome
IBD	Inflammatory bowel disease
ICP	Intracranial pressure
IDDM	Insulin-dependent DM
IGF-1	Insulin-like growth factor-1

IHD	Ischaemic heart disease
IL	Interleukin
IP_3	Inositol 1,4,5-trisphosphate
ITP	Immune thrombocytopenic purpura
IUCD	Intra-uterine contraceptive device
IUGR	Intrauterine growth retardation
IVC	Inferior vena cava
IVF	In vitro fertilisation
IVP	Intravenous pyelogram
JVP	Jugular venous pressure
LDH	Lactate dehydrogenase
LH	Luteinising hormone
LHRH	Luteinising Hormone Releasing Hormone
LMN	Lower motor neurone
LV	Left ventricular
LVH	Left ventricular hypertrophy
MCP	Metacarpophalangeal
MCV	Mean cell volume
MEN	Multiple endocrine neoplasia
MI	Myocardial infarction
MND	Motor neurone disease
MNJ	Neuromuscular junction
MS	Multiple sclerosis
MTP	Metatarsophalangeal
NF	Neurofibromatosis
NIDDM	Non-insulin-dependent DM
NSAIDs	Non-steroidal anti-inflammatory drugs
OCD	Obsessive-compulsive disorder
OCP	Oral contraceptive pill
OGD	Oesophagogastroduodenoscopy
OGTT	Oral glucose tolerance test
PCOS	Poly-cystic ovarian syndrome
PD	Parkinson's disease
PE	Pulmonary embolism
PEFR	Peak expiratory flow rate
PICU	Paediatric intensive care unit
PID	Pelvic inflammatory disease
PIP	Proximal interphalangeal
PAN	Polyarteritis nodosa
PND	Paroxysmal nocturnal dyspnoea

PO	Per os
POP	Progesterone-only pill
PPH	Post-partum haemorrhage
PPIs	Proton pump inhibitors
PR	Per rectum
PRL	Prolactin
PSA	Prostate specific antigen
PTCA	Percutaneous transluminal coronary angioplasty
PTH	Parathyroid hormone
PUO	Pyrexia of unknown origin
RA	Rheumatoid arthritis
RBC	Red blood cell
RF	Rheumatoid factor
RPGN	Rapidly progressive glomerulonephritis
RSV	Respiratory syncytial virus
RUQ	Right upper quadrant
SERM	Selective oestrogen-receptor modulator
SGA	Small for gestational age
SHBG	Sex-hormone-binding globulin
SIADH	Syndrome of inappropriate ADH secretion
SLE	Systemic lupus erythematosus
SOB	Shortness of breath
SVC	Superior vena cava
TB	Tuberculosis
TBG	Thyroxine-binding globulin
TCC	Transitional cell carcinomas
TIA	Transient ischaemic attack
TNF	Tumour necrosis factor
TRH	Thyrotrophin-releasing hormone
TSH	Thyroid-stimulating hormone
TTP	Thrombotic thrombocytopenic purpura
UC	Ulcerative colitis
U&E	Urea and electrolytes
UMN	Upper motor neurone
UTI	Urinary tract infection
VSD	Ventricular septal defect
VZV	Varicella zoster virus
WCC	White cell count
ZIFT	Zygote intrafallopian transfer

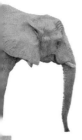

1. Clinical skills

Full medical history

State the following before beginning any history:

- Introduction
- Permission
- How long it will take
- Confidential
- History followed by examination

- Name
- DoB
- Age

Presenting complaint

- 'Can you tell me **when you were last well** and in your own words **what has happened since then?**'
- (Do not interrupt the patient as they talk for at least 2–3 mins, provide appropriate non-verbal cues and show them that you are paying attention).

History of presenting complaint

- 'So you have told me about your illness; can I ask you if you think there was anything that might have **TRIGGERED** the onset of your illness?
- And what has been the **COURSE** of your illness – has it got **better over time, worse over time**, has it **stayed the same**?
- Have there been any periods where you have been **completely free** of the problem?
- Over the course of **24 h** when are you most bothered by your complaint?'

To recall this the mnemonic **OPERATES** may help:

O **O**nset of complaint
P **P**rogress of complaint
E **E**xacerbating factors
R **R**elieving factors
A **A**ssociated symptoms
T **T**iming
E **E**pisodes of being symptom-free
S Relevant **S**ystemic and general inquiry can be added here

Pain history

A pain history can follow a similar format as shown below:

LOTTRAADIO

L **L**ocation
O **O**nset – what were you doing when it started?
T **T**iming – how long did it last?
T **T**ype (sharp/throbbing/gnawing?)
R **R**adiation
A **A**ssociated symptoms (nausea/vomiting/sweating)
A **A**ggravating factors
D **D**ecreasing factors
I **I**ntensity on a scale of 1–10 with 10 being the worst pain imaginable
O **O**ffset – what were you doing when it stopped?

Alternatively: **SOCRATIC**

S **S**ite
O **O**nset – what were you doing when it started?
C **C**haracter (sharp/throbbing/gnawing?)
R **R**adiation
A **A**ssociated symptoms (nausea/vomiting/sweating)
T **T**iming – how long did it last?
I **I**mproving/worsening factors
C **C**ount the pain on a scale of 1–10 with 10 being the most severe pain imaginable

Past medical history

- In hospital before?
- Illnesses? (see MCJ THHREADS)
- Operations?
- Immunisation status?
- Have you ever been abroad?

Risk factors

Most apt for atheromatous disease (mnemonic – **SHAHED** (the co-author of this book))

S **S**moking
H **H**ypertension
A **A**lcohol
H **H**yperlipidaemia
E **E**xercise and healthy **E**ating
D **D**M

MCJ THHREADS

M **M**I
C **C**ancer
J **J**aundice
T **T**B
H **H**ypertension
H **H**ypercholesterolaemia
R **R**heumatic fever as a child
E **E**pilepsy
A **A**sthma
D **D**M
S **S**troke

Medications/allergies

PILLS

P **P**ills, patient taking any?
I **I**njections, eg **I**nsulin/**I**nhalers (as some patients forget to mention when asked about their medications)
LL **ILL**icit drug use
S **S**ensitivities to anything, ie allergies

Family history

- Are your **parents** still with us?
- If not what did they pass away with?
- Do you have any **siblings** with the same illness?
- Have any of your siblings passed away?
- Do you have **children**, do they have anything similar?

Social history

SAADLES

S   **S**moking – pack years? 20/day for 1 year = 1 pack year

A   **A**lcohol within units? 1 unit = ½ pint beer/1 glass wine/1 measure spirit (female 14 units/week = 7 pints lager/male 21 units/week = 10 ½ pints lager)

ADL   **A**ctivities of **D**aily **L**iving – how do you manage with bathing, cooking, cleaning, shopping? This section should also incorporate what *job* the person does and whether their illness could be related to this

E   **E**njoyment activities, ie recreational activities/hobbies

S   **S**ocial support, ie family, neighbours, carers, GP home visits, district nurses, home help, meals on wheels and financial problems

In a respiratory history, it is important to include the following points:

SOD PETe (no offence meant to anyone called Peter!)

S   **S**moking

O   **O**ccupational exposure to various metals, allergens, etc.

D   **D**rugs being used, ie medications such as amiodarone cause pulmonary fibrosis

PET   **PET** exposure, eg cats, pigeons, etc

General enquiries

In every history don't forget to ask about the **4 (FAWR)** non-specific symptoms the patient may exhibit:

F   **F**ever

A   **A**ppetite

W   **W**eight loss (unintentional)

R   **R**educed energy, ie fatigue/lethargy

Functional enquiry

Neurology

HEADS FAINTS

H Headaches?
E Epilepsy inquiry (see Chapter 9, Neurology)?
A Auditory problems?
D Double vision/Dizziness or problems with balance/co-ordination?
S Syncope?
F Faints/muscles Feel weak?
A HAllucinations?
I Intention/resting tremor?
N Numbness?
T Tingling sensation – pins and needles?
S Speech problems/Sphincter disturbance; urinary/bowel?

Cardiology

HEARTS

H Heart beat awareness, ie palpitations?
E OEdema – ankle swelling?
A Angina pain, ie chest pain?
R Rheumatic fever as a child?
T Tiredness?
S Shortness of breath/Syncope?

Respiratory

COSFFS (coughs!)

C Cough/Chest pain?
O Sputum coughed Out, – colour? quantity? haemoptysis?
S Shortness of breath?
F Funny noises on breathing, ie wheeze and stridor?
F Feeling weak, ie lethargy/Fever?
S Speech impaired, ie hoarseness?

Gastroenterology

Work anatomically from entry to exit

Mouth

- Do you have trouble with your teeth?
- Do you have any difficulty chewing your food?
- Do you have difficulty swallowing your food?

Pharynx and oesophagus

- Difficulty in swallowing? (dysphagia)
- Pain on swallowing? (odynophagia)
- Do you have heartburn?

Stomach

- Any nausea or vomiting?
- Is there anything unusual in the vomitus such as bile, blood (haematemesis)?
- Do you have ulcers, relieved or exacerbated by food?

Liver, biliary tract and pancreas

HEPATIC

H	**H**epatitis inquiry, ie been abroad recently, in contact with anyone suffering from this, IV drug use, unprotected sex/anal sex?
E	**E**nlarged breasts in males, ie gynaecomastia?
P	**P**etechiae, ie easy bruising and bleeding?
A	**A**bdominal swelling – **A**scites?
T	**T**oo much alcohol consumption?
I	**I**mpaired glucose tolerance due to decreased pancreatic function hence polyuria, polydipsia and weight loss; DM?
C	**C**onfusion and drowsiness; hepatic encephalopathy/**C**olour change, ie jaundice/**C**olic, ie right upper quadrant/**C**hills, ie fever and rigors?

Small and large bowels

IF A BIT DAMP

I **I**ncreased or decreased frequency of passing motions? (constipated?)

F **F**luid stools? (diarrhoea)

A **A**nal protrusions, piles or prolapse?

B Fresh **B**lood on toilet paper?

I Feeling of **I**ncomplete emptying? (tenesmus)

T **T**arry foul-smelling stools? (melena)

D **D**ifficulty passing stools?

A Is the **A**ppearance of the stools different? (Pale or discoloured stool)

M **M**ucus or slime in stools?

P **P**ain on passing stools?

Renal system

FUN PHISS

F Increased **F**requency of urination

U **U**rgency

N **N**octuria

P **P**olyuria

H **H**esitancy

I **I**ncontinence, urinary/**I**ncomplete emptying of bladder

S **S**tinging on urination?

S **S**omething unusual in the urine, Blood? Discoloration? 'Frothy'?

Musculoskeletal

STABS

S **S**tiffness: morning or evening?

T **T**enderness or pain in muscles or joints?

A **A**ffected joints distribution, ie symmetrical, axial or peripheral?

B **B**ruising or bleeding into joint?

S **S**wellings around joint?

Psychological state

SAD CASE

S **S**uicidal ideations
A **A**nxiety
D **D**ecreased mood/**D**elusions/**D**isordered thought
C Difficulty **C**oncentrating
A **A**uditory or other hallucinations?
S Difficulties **S**leeping
E **E**ating normally?

Physical examination

This must always begin by forming a general impression of the patient and assessing whether any of the following features are evident:

JACCOLT

J **J**aundice
A **A**naemia
C **C**yanosis – peripheral and central
C **C**lubbing
O **O**edema
L **L**ymphadenopathy
T **T**hyroid problem, ie goitre?

For a specific systems examination, the clinical method of choice that is widely adopted may be recalled by the following statement:

I **P**rescribe **P**lenty **A**nalgesics

I **I**nspection
P **P**alpation
P **P**ercussion
A **A**uscultation

(Neurological system follows a different route and this is covered in Chapter 9)

Information organisation

When asked to discuss a particular disease, the following **surgical sieve** is widely regarded as the best way to proceed:

Dressed **I**n a **S**urgeon's **G**own **A** **P**hysician **M**ight **M**ake **P**rogress

D **D**efinition
I **I**ncidence
S **S**ex
G **G**eography
A **A**etiology
P **P**athogenesis
M **M**acroscopic pathology
M **M**icroscopic pathology
P **P**rognosis

This can then be modified slightly to form a **clinical sieve**: '. . . a physician **S**hould **S**ucceed **I**n **T**reatment': **S**ymptoms, **S**igns, **I**nvestigations, **T**reatment.

Similarly, another sieve which allows the causes of a condition to be recalled:

CIMETIDINE

C **C**ongenital
I **I**nfective
M **M**etabolic
E **E**ndocrine
T **T**rauma
I **I**atrogenic
D **D**egenerative
I **I**diopathic
N **N**eoplastic
E **E**verything else, eg drugs

Investigations

The sequence of ordering investigations can be remembered as follows:

Bright **S**tudents **R**emember **S**igns & **S**ymptoms

B　**B**loods – haematology, biochemistry, immunology, etc . . .

S　**S**ecretion samples – sputum, pleural fluid, ascitic fluid, urine, stools, semen, cerebrospinal fluid (CSF), joint aspirate

R　**R**adiology – x-ray, ultrasound scan, CT, MRI, barium studies (swallow, meal, enema)

S　'**S**copes' – oesophagogastroduodenoscopy (OGD), ERCP, bronchoscopy, sigmoidoscopy (rigid and flexible) colonoscopy

S　**S**ample of tissue – biopsy; cytology and histology

Management

As management incorporates all of the above features, ie history-taking, clinical examination, investigations as well as treatment, the treatment of any disease can be classified under the following headings:

Careful **M**anagement **S**hows **P**rogress

C　**C**onservative – ● Lifestyle changes eg stop smoking, reduce alcohol intake, exercise, etc . . .
　　　　　　　　　　　● Input from nurses, physiotherapists, occupational therapists and social services

M　**M**edical –　　　Pharmacological therapy

S　**S**urgical –　　　Operative procedure, interventional radiology

P　**P**alliative –　　Chemotherapy/radiotherapy

NB Whether or not all the above measures are needed to treat a particular condition depends upon each individual case, but this is a general guide to recall the different avenues that can be employed in treatment.

Throughout the book we have not focussed very heavily on the investigation and management side of a condition. Rather, we hope the reader will find the above aide memoires useful and can apply these to all the conditions encountered. Thus, limiting the number of mnemonics needed to learn!

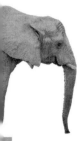

2. Cardiovascular

Histology

Vascular endothelium: simplified cross-section

LIMA

L **L**umen
I **I**ntima
M **M**edia
A **A**dventitia

Anatomy

Heart

Heart valves: order in circuit

TRI before you BI

Tricuspid valve is located between the right atria and right ventricle and the **Bi**cuspid valve is located between the left atria and left ventricle. Blood flows through the **tri**cuspid **before** the **bi**cuspid.

Heart valves: closure sequence

Might **T**ry **A** **P**ull

Mitral
Tricuspid
Aortic
Pulmonic

Heart valve auscultation sites

All **P**atients **T**ake **M**edications

Starting from top left:

Aortic – 2nd intercostal space, right sternal edge
Pulmonary – 2nd intercostal space, left sternal edge
Tricuspid – 4th intercostal space, right sternal edge
Mitral – 5th intercostal space, mid-clavicular line

Apex beat: differential for impalpable apex beat

DOPES (It's not just dopes who can't find it!)

D   **D**extrocardia
O   **O**besity
P   **P**ericarditis/**P**ericardial tamponade/**P**neumothorax
E   **E**mphysema
S   **S**tudent incompetence/**S**coliosis/**S**keletal abnormalities
       (eg pectus excavatum)

Apex beat: abnormalities found on palpation

HILT

H   **H**eaving
I   **I**mpalpable
L   **L**aterally displaced
T   **T**hrusting/**T**apping

Diseases and conditions

Angina pectoris

Definition

ANGI

Acute central chest pain upon exertion due to **N**arrowing of coronary vessels **G**radually limits myocardial blood supply leading to **I**schaemia

Precipitants

4 Es

E **E**xercise
E **E**ating – following meal
E **E**motions
E **E**xposure to cold

Management through alteration in lifestyle

SLEW

S **S**moking cessation
L **L**ow-fat diet
E **E**xercise
W **W**eight loss

Management of acute unstable angina

3 As and BALI

A **A**dmit, bed rest, high-flow oxygen
A **A**nalgesia
A **A**spirin, or clopidogrel if aspirin allergy
B **B**eta blockers
A **A**ngiography with or without angioplasty/CABG if symptoms
    fail to improve
L **L**MW heparin
I **I**nfusion of nitrates

Management of acute stable angina

(Whilst also managing other risk factors such as hypertension,
hyperlipidaemia and diabetes mellitus)

ABC BAGS

A **A**spirin
B **B**eta blockers
C **C**alcium channel blockers
B **B**ypass of coronary arteries if three vessel or left main-stem
    coronary stenosis
A **A**ngioplasty (PTCA) improves symptoms but not mortality
    rates
G **G**TN spray for immediate symptomatic relief
S **S**tatin if total cholesterol >5 mmol/l

Aortic dissection

Aetiology

CHAT

C **C**onnective tissue disease (SLE, RA, Ehlers–Danlos)/
   Congenital cardiovascular anomalies (coarctation of the aorta)
H **H**ypertension (biggest risk factor)
A **A**ortic atherosclerosis/**A**ortitis (eg Takayasu's aortitis, tertiary
   syphilis)
T **T**rauma

Presentation

SCAR

S **S**udden central pain, 'tearing' in nature, may radiate to the
   back
C **C**oronary artery occlusion can lead to chest pain, MI or
   angina pectoris/**C**arotid obstruction can lead to hemiparesis,
   dysphasia or blackouts
A **A**nterior spinal artery can be affected leading to paraplegia
R **R**enal artery can be affected leading to anuria or renal failure

Findings on examination

CHAMP

C **C**ollapsing pulse and an early diastolic murmur above the
   aortic area
H **H**ypertension and a discrepancy in the blood pressure
   between the arms of >20 mmHg
A **A**rm pulses are unequal
M **M**urmur on the back inferior to left scapula, descends to
   abdomen
P **P**alpable abdominal mass (sometimes)

Arrhythmias

Types of arrhythmias

Vague, **B**enign **A**nd **S**ometimes **S**evere
Ventricular tachycardia
Bradycardia
Atrial fibrillation/flutter
Sick sinus syndrome
Supraventricular tachycardia

Bradycardia

Sinus bradycardia, causes

BASHED

B   **B**eta blockers
A   **A**thletes
S   **S**ick-sinus syndrome
H   **H**ypothyroidism
E   **E**lectrolyte imbalance
D   **D**igoxin

Tachycardia

Supraventricular tachycardia: treatment

ABCDE

A   **A**denosine
B   **B**eta blocker
C   **C**alcium channel blocker
D   **D**igoxin
E   **E**xcitation (vagal stimulation)

Wolf–Parkinson–White (WPW) syndrome

WPW

Weird **P**ath**W**ay exists between atria and ventricles and needs to be ablated

Changes on resting ECG

WPW

W **W**ave (Delta) seen in V1
P **P**-R interval is short
W **W**idened QRS complex due to the delta wave

Atrial fibrillation

Causes

SHIMMERS

S **S**oaring BP ie HTN
H **H**eart failure
I **I**schaemic heart disease (**I**HD)
M **M**I
M **M**itral valve disease
E **E**thanol (alcohol)/**E**ndocrine eg thyrotoxicosis
R **R**espiratory causes eg pneumonia, PE, bronchial carcinoma/
     Rheumatic heart disease
S **S**ick sinus syndrome/**S**epsis

Prophylaxis

AF (this is the same as chemical cardioversion)

A **A**miodarone
F **F**lecainide

Management

ABCD

A **A**nti-coagulate
B **B**eta blockers to control rate
C **C**ardiovert/**C**alcium channel blockers
D **D**igoxin

Murmurs

Questions to answer an examination

SCRIPT

S **S**ite
C **C**haracter (eg harsh, soft, blowing)
R **R**adiation
I **I**ntensity
P **P**itch
T **T**iming

Right versus left valves

RIPT + LEAM

RI (Right) **P**ulmonary and **T**ricuspid valves
LE (Left) **A**ortic and **M**itral valves

Right versus left loudness

RILE

Right-sided heart murmurs are loudest on **I**nspiration
Left-sided heart murmurs are loudest on **E**xpiration
Remember **RI**ght and **LE**ft

Aortic stenosis

Causes

REC

R **R**heumatic heart disease
E **E**lderly calcification of a tricuspid aortic valve (the most common)
C **C**ongenital calcification of a bicuspid aortic valve

Presentation

SADDLER

S **S**yncope on exercise
A **A**ngina
D **D**yspnoea
D **D**izziness
L **L**eft heart failure
E **E**mboli from heavily calcified valve = small strokes
R **R**ight heart failure secondary to left heart failure

On examination

PALE PETS

P **P**ulse pressure narrow
A **A**pex beat is not displaced, but is forceful and thrusting in nature (due to LVH)
L **L**eft ventricular outflow obstruction, left ventricular hypertrophy and enlarged coronary arteries
E **E**jection click may be heard from a bicuspid valve
P **P**ulsus alternans
E **E**jection-systolic murmur radiates to the carotids
T **T**hrill palpable in the aortic area
S **S**low rising carotid pulse

Complications

SLAMS

S **S**udden death
L **L**eft ventricular failure
A **A**rrhythmias
M **M**I
S **S**tokes–Adams attacks

Aortic regurgitation

Causes

IM DR CRASH

I	**I**nfective endocarditis
M	**M**arfan's syndrome
D	**D**issection (aortic)
R	**R**heumatic fever
C	**C**ongenital
R	**R**heumatoid arthritis
A	**A**nkylosing spondylitis
S	**S**LE
H	**H**ypertension

Aortic regurgitation (Acute): on examination

WATCH SLAP

W	**W**eakness
A	**A**ngina
T	**T**achycardia
C	**C**yanosis
H	**H**ypotension
S	**S**evere dyspnoea
L	**L**eft ventricular failure
A	**A**ustin–Flint murmur
P	**P**alpitations

Aortic regurgitation (Chronic): on examination

WATCH HEAD UP

W **W**ater-hammer pulse (Corrigan's pulse)/**w**ide pulse pressure
A **A**pex is **displaced and hyperdynamic**
T **T**raube's sign (pistol shot over femoral arteries)
C **C**arotid pulsation (Corrigan's sign)/**C**apillary pulsation in nail bed (Quincke's sign)
H **H**ead-nodding (De Musset's sign)
H **H**ill sign – systolic pressure in the lower extremity is raised in comparison to higher extremity by >100 mmHg
E **E**asily missed decrescendo diastolic murmur
A **A**ustin–Flint murmur
D **D**uroziez's sign – systolic–diastolic murmur produced by compressing femoral artery with stethoscope
U **U**vula has pulsation – Muller's sign
P **P**upils have pulsations – Becker's sign

Mitral stenosis

Causes

CRAP

C **C**ongenital
R **R**heumatic
A **A**ND
P **P**rosthetic valve

Presentation

MALAR PATCHES

M **M**alar flush (cheeks)
A **A**trial fibrillation is common
L **L**eft heart failure
A **A**pex beat is tapping, undisplaced
R **R**ight heart failure

P **P**alpitations
A **A**uscultation (loud S1 with an opening snap and a rumbling mid-diastolic murmur heard best with patient on their left side and in expiration; a Graham–Steell murmur is sometimes found)
T **T**hromboembolism may be the first symptom
C **C**achexia/**C**yanosis/**COPD or C**hronic bronchitis-like scenario especially if left main bronchus is compressed causing bronchiectasis
H **H**aemoptysis, rupture of congested bronchioles/**H**oarse voice (massive enlargement of left atrium)
E **E**mboli (systemic) risk of hemiplegia/ patient in sinus rhythm is at risk of embolism
S **S**yncope

Mitral regurgitation

Causes

IF CREEP

I **I**nfective endocarditis
F **F**unctional (LV dilatation)
C **C**ardiomyopathy/**C**ongenital
R **R**heumatic fever/**R**uptured chordae tendinae
E **E**lderly calcification
E **E**hlers–Danlos syndrome
P **P**apillary muscle dysfunction/rupture

Presentation

AFRAID PA

A **A**F
F **F**atigue
R **R**ight ventricular heave
A **A**pex is displaced and hyperdynamic
I **I**nfective endocarditis
D **D**yspnoea
P **P**alpitations
A **A**uscultation reveals soft S1 and splitting of S2 with a loud P2 (pulmonary hypertension) and a pansystolic murmur at apex which radiates to the axilla

Mitral stenosis (MS) versus regurgitation (MR): epidemiology

MS is a female title (**Ms**) and it is female predominant
MR is a male title (**Mr**) and it is male predominant

Cardiac arrest

Aetiology

4 Hs, 4 Ts

H **H**ypoxia
H **H**ypothermia
H **H**ypo-**h**yperkalaemia
H **H**ypovolaemia
T **T**amponade (cardiac)
T **T**ension pneumothorax
T **T**hromboembolism
T **T**oxins

Management, Basic Life Support (BLS)

ABC

A **A**irway, clear and maintain with chin lift/jaw thrust/head tilt (if no spinal injury)
B **B**reathing, look, listen and feel, if not breathing give two life saving breaths immediately
C **C**irculation, carotid pulse for at least 10 s, if absent give 15 chest compressions at 100/min

Continue the cycle of 2 breaths and 15 compressions and check the circulation every minute, proceed to more advanced life support when possible.

Management, Advanced Life Support (ALS)

CDE (with A after every step)

C **C**ardiac monitor and defibrillator should be attached to the patient
A **A**ssess rhythm and pulse
D **D**efibrillate × 3 if VF or pulseless VT, CPR for 1 min
A **A**ssess rhythm and pulse
E **E**MD (no cardiac output despite ECG showing electrical activity) or asystole warrants CPR for 3 min
A **A**ssess rhythm and pulse

During CPR

Check **PEC** and attempt **AEIO**

P **P**addle positions
E **E**lectrode
C **C**ontacts

A **A**drenaline
E **E**ndotracheal intubation
I **I**V access
O **O**xygen (high-flow)

Cardiac failure

Definition

Cardiac output **fails** to meet body's needs, despite normal venous pressures

JVP elevation: causes

SHOT

S **S**upraclavicular lymphatic enlargement
H **H**eart failure (right)
O **O**bstruction of vena cava – supraclavicular
T Intra-**T**horacic pressure increase

Left heart failure

Aetiology

I MACH

I **I**HD
M **M**itral regurgitation
A **A**ortic valve disease
C **C**ardiomyopathy
H **H**ypertension

Symptoms

Symptoms are caused by pulmonary congestion

PC FOWD

P **P**aroxysmal nocturnal dyspnoea
C **C**ough
F **F**atigue
O **O**rthopnoea
W **W**heeze
D **D**yspnoea

On examination

MAT the **CAT**

M **M**urmur, pansystolic (functional mitral regurgitation)
A **A**pex beat is displaced
T **T**achycardia
C **C**rackles (bilateral, basal)
A **A**uscultation reveals 3rd heart sound (Gallop rhythm; rapid ventricular filling)
T **T**achypnoea

Right heart failure

Aetiology

PC SPITE

P **P**ulmonary valve disease
C **C**ardiomyopathy
S **S**econdary to left heart failure
P **P**ericardial tamponade
I **I**nfarction
T **T**ricuspid regurgitation
E **E**mbolism (pulmonary)

Symptoms

FACIAL PAN

F **F**atigue
A **A**nkles swollen
C **C**erebral signs (faints/headaches)
I **I**ncreased urinary frequency
A **A**norexia
L **L**iver congestion (mild jaundice/coagulation problems)
P **P**alpitations
A **A**scites
N **N**ausea

On examination

PJ HAT

P **P**itting ankle/sacral oedema
J **J**VP is raised
H **H**epatomegaly
A **A**scites
T **T**ricuspid regurgitation signs

Chest X-ray changes of heart failure

ABCDE

A **A**lveolar oedema (peri-hilar shadowing; 'bats wings')
B Kerley **B**-lines (interstitial oedema)
C **C**ardiomegaly (heart > 50% of thoracic width)
D **D**ilated prominent upper lobe vessels
E Pleural **E**ffusion

Heart failure: management

BAD IV

B   **B**eta-blockers
A   **A**CE inhibitors
D   **D**iuretics
I   **I**notropes (digoxin)
V   **V**asodilators

Heart failure: causes of exacerbation

FAILURE

F   **F**orgot medication
A   **A**rrhythmia/**A**naemia
I   **I**scheamia/**I**nfarction/**I**nfection
L   **L**ifestyle: taken too much salt
U   **U**pregulation of cardiac output: pregnancy, hyperthyroidism
R   **R**enal failure
E   **E**mbolism (pulmonary)

Pulmonary oedema

Management

SMINT

S   **S**it up and give high-flow oxygen via face mask
M   **M**orphine (+ **m**etoclopramide)
I   **I**V diuretic (furosemide)
N   **N**itrate (GTN) spray/IV
T   **T**ailor further management to ensure adequate ventilation and gas exchange and correct haemodynamic disturbance

Cardiomyopathy

Definition

Cardio**myo**pathy: disease of the **myo**cardium. Can be divided into three categories: dilated, hypertrophic or restrictive

Dilated cardiomyopathy (DCM)

Aetiology

HIP FACT

H **H**aemochromatosis
I **I**diopathic (majority of cases)
P **P**ostviral myocarditis
F **F**amilial
A **A**lcohol
C **C**ocaine
T **T**hyrotoxicosis

Signs and symptoms

A DAFT HIT

A **A**rrhythmias
D **D**eath (sudden)
A **A**pex beat is displaced
F **F**unctional mitral and tricuspid regurgitations
T **T**hromboembolism
H **H**eart failure symptoms
I **I**ncreased JVP
T **T**hird heart sound

Hypertrophic obstructive cardiomyopathy (HOCM)

Aetiology

GI

G **G**enetic
I **I**diopathic

Signs and symptoms

A SAD ACE

A **A**ngina
S **S**yncope
A **A**rrhythmias
D **D**eath (sudden, more common in young patients)
A **A**pex beat is double
C **C**arotid pulse is jerky
E **E**jection systolic murmur

Restrictive cardiomyopathy (RCM)

Aetiology

HI SEA

H	**H**aemochromatosis
I	**I**diopathic
S	**S**arcoidosis
E	**E**ndomyocardial fibrosis
A	**A**myloidosis

Signs and symptoms

SOFIA HAT

S	**S**welling in abdomen
O	**O**edema in ankles
F	**F**atigue
I	**I**ncreased JVP
A	**A**rrhythmias/**A**pex beat palpable
H	**H**epatomegaly
A	**A**scites
T	**T**hird heart sound

Cardiac surgery

Coronary artery bypass graft: indications

STUD

S	**S**tenosis of the left main stem
T	**T**riple vessel disease
U	**U**nstable angina
D	**D**epressed ventricular function

Drugs

Anti-arrhythmics: for AV nodes

Do **B**lock **AV**

D	**D**igoxin
B	**B**eta blockers
A	**A**denosine
V	**V**erapamil

Amiodarone: action, side-effects

6 Ps

P   **P**rolongs action potential duration
P   **P**hotosensitivity
P   **P**igmentation of skin
P   **P**eripheral neuropathy
P   **P**ulmonary alveolitis and fibrosis
P   **P**eripheral conversion of T4 to T3 is inhibited, leading to hypothyroidism

Beta blockers: main contraindications, cautions

ABCDE

A   **A**sthma
B   **B**lock (heart block)
C   **C**OPD
D   **D**iabetes mellitus
E   **E**lectrolyte (hyperkalaemia)

Ca^{2+} channel blockers: uses

CHASM

C   **C**erebral vasospasm/**C**HF
H   **H**ypertension
A   **A**ngina
S   **S**upraventricular tachyarrhythmia
M   **M**igraine

Clopidogrel: use

CLOPIdogrel is a drug that prevents **CL**ots, an **O**ral **P**latelet **I**nhibitor (**OPI**)

HMG-CoA reductase inhibitors (statins): side effects, contraindications

HMG

● Side-effects:

H   **H**epatotoxicity
M   **M**yositis (aka rhabdomyolysis)

● Contraindications:

G   **G**irl during pregnancy/**G**rowing children

Thrombolytic agents

USA

U **U**rokinase
S **S**treptokinase
A **A**lteplase (tPA)

Contraindications to thrombolysis

ABCDEFGHI

A **A**ortic aneurysm
B **B**leeding disorder
C **C**erebrovascular accident; haemorrhagic
D **D**uodenal/gastric ulcer
E **E**xternal chest compression
F **F**lorid liver/renal disease
G **G**ravid uterus
H **H**ypertension (severe uncontrolled ≥180/110 mmHg)
I **I**njury (major trauma/surgery within 1 month)/**I**nternal bleeding (excluding menses)

Heart disease

Atherosclerosis

Risk factors

MR SHAHED (the co-author of this book)

M **M**ale gender
R **R**ace
S **S**moking
H **H**ypertension
A **A**ge – middle-aged, elderly
H **H**yperlipidaemia
E **E**xercise and healthy **E**ating ↓↓
D **D**iabetes mellitus

Hypertension

Endocrine causes of secondary hypertension

CHAP

C   **C**ushing's syndrome
H   **H**yperaldosteronism (aka Conn's syndrome)
A   **A**cromegaly
P   **P**haeochromocytoma

Note: only 5% of hypertension cases are secondary, the rest are primary

Treatment

ABCD

A   **A**CE inhibitors/**A**ngiotensin-II-antagonists (sometimes **A**lpha agonists also)
B   **B**eta blockers
C   **C**alcium channel blockers
D   **D**iuretics (Thiazides)

MI

Symptoms

CUBE

C   **C**entral, crushing chest pains lasting >20 min, radiates to left arm or jaw
U   **U**pset stomach with nausea and vomiting
B   **B**reathlessness
E   **E**xcessive sweating

Management

MAN BOTH

M   **M**orphine
A   **A**spirin
N   **N**itrates
B   **B**eta blockers (if not contraindicated)
O   **O**xygen
T   **T**hrombolytics
H   **H**eparin

Or

MONA

M **M**orphine
O **O**xygen
N **N**itrates
A **A**spirin

Complications

DEPARTS

D **D**eath (sudden)/**D**ressler's syndrome
E **E**mboli (thromboembolism)
P **P**ericarditis
A **A**rrhythmia (ventricular)/**A**neurysm (ventricular)
R **R**upture (myocardial or septal)
T **T**amponade
S **S**hock (cardiogenic)

Pericardial diseases

Pericarditis

Causes

DR IS TRUMP

D **D**ressler's syndrome
R **R**adiotherapy
I **I**nfection (viruses, bacteria, fungi)
S **S**LE
T **T**B
R **R**heumatoid arthritis
U **U**raemia
M **M**alignancy
P **P**ost MI (24–48 h)

Findings

PERICarditis

P   **P**ulsus paradoxus
E   **E**CG changes (saddle-shaped ST segment)
R   **R**ub
I   **I**ncreased JVP
C   **C**hest pain (worse on inspiration, better when lean forwards)

Beck's triad (cardiac tamponade)

3 Ds

D   **D**istant heart sounds
D   **D**istended jugular veins
D   **D**ecreased arterial pressure

Shock

Signs and symptoms

TORCHES

T   **T**achycardia
O   **O**liguria/multi-**O**rgan damage
R   **R**espiration shallow/rapid
C   **C**ool skin/**C**yanotic
H   **H**ypotension
E   **E**yes blank/**E**levated JVP or reduced
S   **S**ympathetic response – vomiting, anxious, sweating

Miscellaneous

ECG: left bundle branch block (LBBB) vs. right bundle branch block (RBBB)

WiLLiaM MoRRoW

W pattern of QRS in V1–V2 and **M** pattern of QRS in V3–V6 is **L**BBB

M pattern of QRS in V1–V2 and **W** pattern of QRS in V3–V6 is **R**BBB

Note: consider bundle branch blocks when QRS complex is wide

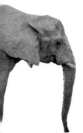

3. Clinical chemistry

Aspirin

Aspirin overdose

Aetiology

SAD

S   **S**uicidal attempt
A   **A**ccident
D   **D**eliberate self-harm

Reye's syndrome, symptoms

LAD

Even small amounts of aspirin ingestion can lead to toxicity in adults, whilst even smaller doses put children at risk of developing Reye's syndrome

L   **L**iver disturbances
A   **A**cidosis (metabolic)
D   **D**isturbed CNS

Early symptoms

DAFT HID

D   **D**eafness
A   **A**ppear flushed
F   **F**ever
T   **T**innitus
H   **H**yperventilation
I   **I**ncreased sweating
D   **D**izziness

Late symptoms

HEFT

H   **H**yperventilation
E   **E**pigastric tenderness
F   **F**ever
T   **T**achycardia

Pathology

Had **A** **C**up, **D**estroyed **H**er **M**etabolism

H   **H**yperventilation is caused by aspirin due to stimulation of
the CNS respiratory centre which increases respiratory rate
and depth
A   **A**lkalosis (respiratory) results from hyperventilation
C   **C**ompensation by the body by increasing urinary bicarbonate
and potassium excretion which leads to . . .
D   **D**ehydration and . . .
H   **H**ypokalaemia, which can result in . . .
M   **M**etabolic acidosis

Hyperlipidaemia

Aetiology

It is divided into primary and secondary

- **Primary**, most have unknown aetiologies
- **Secondary**, divided into increased levels of triglycerides and
  increased levels of cholesterol

Increased levels of triglycerides

Aetiology

CHAN

C   **C**holestatic liver disease
H   **H**ypothyroidism
A   **A**norexia nervosa
N   **N**ephrotic syndrome

Increased levels of cholesterol

Aetiology

ADD HOC

A **A**lcohol
D **D**M
D **D**rugs
H **H**epatocellular diseases
O **O**besity
C **C**hronic renal disease

Signs

Most of the signs can be divided into signs of complications and signs of lipid deposition

Signs of complications

CAP

C **C**arotid bruit
A **A**ssociated high BP
P **P**eripheral pulses are decreased

Signs of lipid deposition

ELECT

E **E**yes, around them (xanthelasma)
L **L**ipidaemia retinalis (pale retinal vessels)
E **E**lbows and knees (tuberous xanthomas)
C **C**orneal arcus
T **T**endon xanthomas (Achilles tendon, extensor tendons of hands, patella tendon)

HDL versus LDL

HDL is **H**ealthy, cardioprotective, transports lipids to the liver

LDL is **L**azy, taken up by macrophages and forms atheromatous plaque

Paracetamol

Paracetamol overdose

The most common intentional drug overdose in the UK

Risk factors

COMAH

C **C**hronic alcohol abusers
O **O**n drugs that increase cytochrome P450 activity, anti-TB
drugs
M **M**alnourished individuals
A **A**norexics
H **H**IV patients

Time course of signs and symptoms

MS REEJ

1st 24 h

M **M**ild nausea, lethargy, malaise and vomiting
S **S**igns are not evident at this early stage

24–36 h

R **R**UQ pain, vomiting
E **E**nlarged liver which is tender

36–72 h

E **E**ncephalopathy (confusion) increases, jaundice
J **J**aundice, coagulopathy, renal pain and hypoglycaemia

Pathogenesis

A small proportion of paracetamol is always metabolised by
cytochrome P450 to a highly reactive intermediate
N-acetyl-*P*-benzoquinoneimine (NAPQI) which is activated by
conjugation with glutathione.

Patterns of acute liver necrosis

CL

Centrilobular pattern seen in moderate damage, **L**obular pattern seen in severe damage. Remember **L** comes after **C** in the alphabet and is therefore a furtherance of the damage.

Complications

CHAMP

C **C**erebral oedema
H **H**ypoglycaemia
A **A**cute hepatic failure
M **M**etabolic acidosis
P **P**ancreatitis

Metabolic acidosis

Causes

UK SLAMS

U **U**raemia
K **K**etoacidosis
S **S**alicylates
L **L**actic acidosis
A **A**lcohol
M **M**ethanol
S **S**epsis

Hypokalaemia

Features

IT MIMICS PHD

I	Increases paralytic ileus (aggravates)
T	Tetany
M	Muscle weakness
I	Increases possibility of hepatic encephalopathy
M	Muscle cramps
I	Increases PR interval, T wave and prominent U wave
C	Cardiac arrhythmias
S	ST segment depression
P	Polyuria
H	Hypotonia
D	Digoxin toxicity

Causes

ADD CLIP

Alkalosis
Diuretics
Diarrhoea and vomiting
Cushing's syndrome/Conn's syndrome
Laxative abuse
Intestinal fistulae
Pyloric stenosis

Hyperkalaemia

Causes

WEAKER

W	Whack – ie tissue injury (burns), rhabdomyolysis
E	Extracting blood whilst fist is clenched/Excess K^+ therapy
A	ACE inhibitors/metabolic Acidosis/Addison's disease
K	K-sparing diuretics
E	Exchange of blood massive (ie massive blood transfusion)
R	Renal failure (oliguric)

ECG changes of hyperkalaemia

Although not a mnemonic it is a favourite question for clinical and written papers.

i.   Flat P waves
ii. Broad bizarre QRS complexes
iii. Slurred ST segment
iv. Tall tented T waves
v.   U wave follows the T waves

Management of hyperkalaemia

C BIG

C   **C**alcium gluconate/**C**alcium resonium
B   **B**icarbonate
I   **I**nsulin
G   **G**lucose

Hyponatraemia

Causes

KILLER (can be if left untreated!)

K   **K**idney disease – renal failure, nephrotic syndrome
I   **I**atrogenic – diuretics especially thiazides
L   **L**iver disease – cirrhosis
L   **L**oss of fluid – diarrhoea, vomiting, dehydration
E   **E**ndocrine disease – SIADH, hypothyroidism, adrenal insufficiency (Addison's disease)
R   **R**educed cardiac output – cardiac failure

Hypernatraemia

Causes

ARID (because they present with thirst)

A **A**ldosterone increase
R **R**enal disease
I **I**atrogenic; diuretics (ie mannitol)/excessive saline
D **D**iabetes insipidus

Or

The 4 Ds

D **D**iuretics
D **D**ehydration
D **D**iabetes insipidus
D **D**iarrhoea

Hypocalcaemia

Causes

HAM

H **H**ypoparathyroidism (the most important cause, often follows thyroidectomy)
A **A**cute pancreatitis
M **M**alnutrition/**M**alfunctioning of kidneys ie chronic renal failure

Features

TAP CT

T **T**etany
A **A**bdominal cramps
P **P**erioral paraesthesia
C **C**hvosteck's sign (**tapping** on facial nerve causes facial spasm)
T **T**rousseau's sign (carpal spasm after occlusion with sphygmomanometer)

Hypercalcaemia

Causes

CHAMPS

C **C**alcium supplementation/**C**ancers eg myeloma, bone metastases
H **H**yperparathyroidsim (1°)
A **A**ddison's disease/**A**cromegaly
M **M**ilk-alkali syndrome
P **P**aget's disease
S **S**arcoidosis and other granulomatous disease

Features

Bones, stones, groans and psychic moans
Bones (may present with fractures)
Stones (kidney stones)
Groans (abdominal groans, anorexia and constipation)
Psychic moans (weakness and fatigue with altered mental state)

Increased anion gap

Causes

ASIDE (it moves aside)

A **A**cidosis (lactic)
S **S**alicylates
I **I**ntoxication
D **D**KA
E **E**thylene glycol

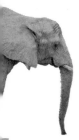

4. Dermatology

Many disorders directly affect the skin and many systemic disorders have dermatological manifestations. A few dermatological conditions have the potential to become life threatening, but other skin conditions can make life distressing for the individual.

Skin

Functions of skin

SKIN

S **S**pecialised sensory innervation/**S**ynthesise Vitamin D/ **S**ecretes pheromones for **S**ex
K **K**eeps out unwanted molecules, microbes or radiation/**K**eeps in water, electrolytes and solutes
I **I**mmunological function; contains antigen-presenting cells
N **N**ormalises heat regulation

Dermatology anatomy and histology

The skin has three layers

EDF

E **E**pidermis
D **D**ermis
F **F**at

Epidermis

Skin **M**ay **L**ike **M**oisturiser **B**ut . . .

S   **S**tratified epithelium (keratinocytes)
M   **M**elanocytes
L   **L**angerhans cells
M   **M**erkel's cells
B   **B**asal lamina (secures epidermis to dermis)

Dermis

Face **C**reams **E**specially **G**ood **B**ecause **L**ook **N**ice

F   **F**ibrous tissue
C   **C**ollagen
E   **E**lastin
G   **G**lycosaminoglycans
B   **B**lood vessels
L   **L**ymphatic vessels
N   **N**eural elements (sweat glands, sebaceous glands, hair follicles)

Diseases and conditions

Acne rosacea

Clinical presentation

ROSACEA

R   **R**elapsing remitting facial disorder
O   **O**ften precedes the development of fixed erythema (chin, nose, cheeks, forehead)
S   **S**welling and soft tissue overgrowth of the nose (rhinophyma) may occur
A   **A**void excessive sun exposure
C   **C**hronic flushing triggered by spicy food, alcohol and high emotion
E   **E**ye problems are commonly blepharitis, conjunctivitis, keratitis
A   **A**ntibiotics used during flare ups

Acne vulgaris

Clinical presentation

ACNE.V

A **A**dolescents mostly affected by acne vulgaris/**A**ffects face, upper chest and back

C **C**omedone (blackhead) is main problem

N **N**ormal skin commensal, *Propionibacterium acnes*, thrives in blocked follicles, inflammatory response to their presence causes the angry, red appearance of inflamed lesions

E **E**xcessive sebum production occurs under the control of androgens

V **V**ariety of skin presentations, including: comedones, red papules, pustules, nodules, cysts

Blistering disorders (pemphigoid/pemphigus)

PemphiGoid, due to IgG autoantibodies against parts of the basement membrane

Basal cell carcinoma (rodent ulcer)

Clinical presentation

RODENT

R **R**olled telangiectactic edge around the nodule

O **O**ften found on the face

D **D**estructive locally if untreated

E **E**xcision is best for small lesions

N **N**odule is pearly

T **T**endency to occur in fair-skinned

Eczema and dermatitis

The terms are sometimes used interchangeably. Dermatitis often refers to an eczema of external origin

Atopic eczema

ATOPIC

A **A**llergens, such as animal dander, aggravate eczema
T **T**reatment of skin dryness with daily use of emollients, especially greasy emollients. Topical steroids required in active eczema (red, painful, weeping and itchy)
O **O**veruse of topical steroids in children can lead to skin thinning, striae and adrenal suppression
P **P**arents with an IL4 receptor mutation are often found in children with atopic eczema
I **I**nfection with *Staphylococcus aureus* is found in many patients
C **C**hildren often grow out of eczema

Contact dermatitis

Common allergens for allergic contact dermatitis

CONTACT

C **C**utaneous type IV reaction
O **O**intments and cosmetics containing lanolin
N **N**ickel
T **T**opical antibiotics can cause it, ie neomycin
A **A**utosensitisation can occur (secondary spread elsewhere)
C **C**hromates (cement, leather)/**C**olophony (plasters, glues, inks)
T **T**opical antihistamines and topical anaesthetics (haemorrhoid creams) can cause it

The worsening of symptoms in irritant dermatitis

RaW DaFt

R **R**ed
W **W**eep
D **D**ry
F **F**issure

Seborrhoeic dermatitis

Clinical presentation of adult seborrhoeic dermatitis

SEBORRH

S **S**caly eruption of unknown aetiology

E **E**yebrows can be affected

B **B**ased around face and head, on scalp causes dandruff, also found on nasolabial folds, cheeks and flexures

O **O**vergrowth of yeasts in skin could be a cause

R **R**esponds to mild topical steroids and antifungal preparations

R **R**ed in colour but can have a yellowish appearance

H **H**IV-positive individuals can be affected quite severely

Haemangiomas

Haemangiomas (strawberry naevus/pyogenic granuloma)

STRAW

S **S**mall red spot

T **T**ypically occurs in infants in first few months of life

R **R**apidly enlarges over following few months

A **A**rrest in growth occurs for unknown reason

W **W**ill spontaneously involute by the age of 5–7, no treatment needed

Drug eruptions

Urticaria

DURTICARIA

D **D**irect mast cell degranulation
U **U**sually lasts from minutes to a few hours
R **R**ed wheals with pale centres are very itchy (**U**rticaria **U**rts!)
T **T**ransfusion of blood products and foreign proteins is common cause
I **I**ngestion of certain drugs leads to rapid onset of this condition
C **C**odeine, morphine and other opioids
A **A**ngioedema may occur
R **R**aised weals
I **I**mmunological and non-immunological mechanisms can cause urticaria
A **A**naphylaxis may occur

Reaction to penicillins

PENEC

P **P**apules are red and particularly affect the trunk along with erythema
E **E**xanthematous/maculopapular reaction
N **N**umber 1 type of cutaneous drug eruption
E **E**osinophilia and fever may occur
C **C**ephalosporins, penicillins and anti-epileptics are the cause

Infestations

Impetigo

Clinical presentation

IMPETIGO

I Infection with *Staphylococcus aureus, Streptococcus pyogenes* or both
M Mostly in young children
P Particularly around nose and surrounding parts of face
E Erythematous base with honey-coloured crusts
T Treat with Topical antibiotic such as fusidic acid for localised lesions
I Individuals are highly contagious from skin-to-skin contact; Improve hygiene; do not share towels
G Gram stain and culture of swab diagnostic
O Oral flucloxacillin required for widespread impetigo

Staphylococcal scalded skin syndrome

SCALD

S Staphylococcal toxins cause Split in superficial epidermis
C Children especially infants are most susceptible
A A few days after initial infection there is sudden onset of widespread tender erythema and fever
L Layers of skin begin to detach in sheets
D Differential diagnosis is toxic epidermal necrolysis due to drugs

Cellulitis

SPREAD

S Subcutaneous infection
P Portal of entry usually obvious (leg ulcer or wound)
R Red tender swelling
E Erysipelas presents very similarly and can be difficult to differentiate from cellulitis
A group A streptococci usually the infection
D Defined edge of spreading erythematous oedema and vesiculation of erysipelas is absent

Necrotising fasciitis

FASCITIS

F   Deep **F**ascia and vessels within it are affected
A   Group **A** streptococci are usually causative
S   **S**econdary death of overlying **S**kin occurs
C   **C**ellulitis-like appearance until 2 days into condition when lesion becomes purplish, haemorrhagic bullae appear and tissue becomes necrotic
I   **I**nsufficient arteries and diabetes mellitus predispose to development but does occur in healthy individuals also
T   **T**reatment is by urgent debridement and high-dose IV benzylpenicillin
I   **I**f untreated there is high mortality
S   **S**kin loss is usually permanent

Clinical presentation of fungal skin infections

FUNGI

F   **F**ungi are eukaryotes with a rigid polysaccharide cell wall
U   **U**sual sites affected are groins (tinea cruris), feet (tinea pedis), nails (tinea unguium)/**U**sually **U**nilateral
N   **N**ormal appearance is of well-defined red lesions with peripheral scale and central clearing
G   Five **G**eneras are important for skin mycoses
I   **I**tchy, **I**nflamed fissured spaces that are moist

Candidiasis

ALBICANS

A   *Candida **A**lbicans* yeast is a common commensal in the gastrointestinal tract, mouth and vagina but not on the skin
L   **L**ocally acting agents should be utilised, such as nystatin, amphotericin B and imidazoles
B   **B**road-spectrum antibiotics can cause candidiasis
I   **I**nvades living tissue unlike dermatophytes
C   *Candida albicans* is the cause in most but not all human cases
A   **A**ngular stomatitis occurs in folds of the mouth usually due to poor fitting dentures
N   **N**ails as well as **N**ailfolds tend to be infected
S   **S**erious systemic infection can occur with *Candida* infection

Viral skin infection, warts

WARTS

W **W**idespread and commonly seen in children, young adults and the immunosuppressed

A **A**etiology is HPV infection of keratinocytes

R **R**esolve naturally in most cases

T **T**opical salicylic acid paints (keratolytic) or cryotherapy can be used to treat

S **S**tubborn lesions occasionally removed with intralesional bleomycin ±lasers

Plantar warts

FEET

F **F**requently resistant to repeated treatments

E **E**xcision is best avoided because they are very infective

E **E**xpect school children to wear verruca socks for swimming

T **T**reat with salicylic acid and cover with a waterproof plaster or try cryotherapy

Molluscum contagiosum (pox virus)

POCS

P **P**ink **P**apules have umbilicated central area

O **O**btain a white cheesy material from the papule and microscope to confirm diagnosis

C **C**ommon in **C**hildren, **C**ontagious and **C**aused by pox virus

S **S**pontaneously resolve

Herpes simplex infection

SIMPLE

S Subclinical primary infection
I Infection is often recurrent and affects genital or perioral areas
M Manifests most commonly as gingivostomatitis
P Painful vesicles are grouped on erythematous base and heal without scarring
L Light, fevers and emotional stress are triggers and at this stage aciclovir can be used to prevent or reduce severity of recurrence
E Evidence that Bell's palsy may be related to recurrent herpes infection

Herpes zoster infection (shingles)

HERPES.Z

H Herpes zoster must be differentiated from Herpes simplex
E Eruption is polymorphic (red papules, vesicles, pustules and crusting)
R Recurrent infection is dermatomal in distribution, one or more dermatomes
P Primary infection is chickenpox
E Eruption may be preceded by symptoms of pain and malaise
S Scarring may occur with healing
Z Varicella Zoster virus becomes dormant in the dorsal root ganglia

Lichen planus

PLANUS

P **P**urple papules are flat-topped and itchy
L **L**acy markings on the surface of the eruption are known as Wickham's striae
A **A**etiology is unknown, hepatitis C virus infection?
N **N**ormally occurs at sites of trauma and affects flexor aspects of the wrists, forearms, ankles and legs. Affects scalp (scarring alopecia), nails (longitudinal ridges), genitals (annular lesions), mouth (on inner cheeks)
U **U**sually persists for 16–18 months
S **S**ymptomatic treatment, topical **S**teroids are used for severe itch

Arthropod skin infection, Scabies

SCABIES

S **S**aliva/faeces of female *Sarcoptes scabiei* mites causes scabies
C **C**lose **C**ontact promotes spread, especially amongst members of a family
A **A**ffects spaces between fingers, wrist flexures, axillae, abdomen especially around umbilicus, buttocks and groin (itchy red penile or scrotal papules are diagnostic)
B **B**urrows in the skin can be scraped and scabies mites extracted and visualised microscopically
I **I**nfants often have affected palms and soles
E **E**ruption is **E**xcoriated and often becomes **E**czematised
S **S**cabies can be treated with an anti-**S**cabetic such as malathion or permethrin

Malignant melanoma

Clinical presentation

MALIGNANT

M **M**alignant melanomas develop from pre-existing **M**oles in 30% of cases

A **A**dults who develop a new mole that is greater than 6 mm in diameter should seek medical advice

L **L**ocal changes include inflammation, crusting, bleeding and sensory changes

I **I**rregular outline of mole from a previously round or oval lesion is cause for concern

G **G**rowing

N **N**on-uniform colour of mole with different shades of brown/black/red or blue is suggestive of malignant melanoma

A **A**ltered size/shape/colour of pre-existing lesion suggests malignant melanoma

N **N**aevi/moles are the clinical differential diagnosis of malignant melanoma in young people

T **T**runks of people older than 50 years frequently have seborrhoeic keratoses

Psoriasis

Clinical presentation

PSORIASIS

P **P**laques are well defined

S **S**ymmetrical plaques

O **O**nycholysis (distal separation from the nail bed) may occur in nails; **O**ccurs in 2% of the UK population

R **R**ed plaques

I **I**nflammatory skin condition; it is **I**mmunologically mediated; TH1-cells predominate in early lesions

A **A**rthropathy develops in 7% of psoriatics

S **S**ilvery scale on plaques on extensor aspects of elbows, knees, **S**calp and **S**acrum

I **I**n young patients very small plaques or guttate are seen, pustular variants are seen on the **p**alms and **s**oles (**p**ustules **s**terile)

S **S**kin is treated with phototherapy (narrow-band UVB TL-01)

Squamous cell carcinoma

Clinical presentation

S,CELL,C

S **S**un-exposed areas are usually affected: ears, dorsum of the hands, bald scalp

C **C**rusted, firm, irregular lesion

E **E**xcision used as treatment

L **L**ower lip can be affected in smokers

L **L**ess likely to metastasise

C Associated with **C**hronic inflammation such as venous leg ulcers

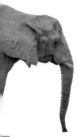

5. Endocrinology

The physiology of hormone synthesis and action

The field of endocrinology is so named because hormones act in a classically endocrine way by exerting effects on a target organ at a distance from the endocrine cell by secretion into the bloodstream. Additionally, some hormones exert paracrine effects on adjacent cells or may also act as neurotransmitters.

Hormone action through cell surface receptors

This occurs through at least three ways. They can be recalled by the '**feline**' mnemonics.

Actions mediated by adenylate cyclase

When adenylate cyclase is activated it generates cyclic AMP (cAMP) as a second messenger. Hormones which act in part or totally via cAMP can be recalled as follows:

CAT FLAP

C **c**AMP (hormone action mediated via)
A **A**CTH
T **T**SH
F **F**SH
L **L**H
A **A**DH
P **P**TH

Actions mediated by phosphatidyl inositols and calcium transport

They do so by inducing the transport or release of calcium with or without the cleavage of cell membrane phospholipids to generate inositol 1,4,5-trisphosphate (IP_3) and diacylglycerol (DG). This information can be remembered as follows:

CAT LID

C **C**alcium transport (hormone action mediated via)
A **A**DH
T **T**RH
L **L**H
I **I**P$_3$ (hormone action mediated via)
D **D**G (hormone action mediated via)

Actions mediated by tyrosine kinase activity

They can be remembered as such:

KITI

K **K**inase (hormone action mediated via)
I **I**nsulin
T **T**yrosine
I **I**GF-1 (hormone action mediated via)

The circulation and subsequent metabolism of hormones

Circulating binding proteins and albumin help prevent steroid and thyroid hormones from being degraded by the liver. The circulating binding proteins help maintain blood hormone levels at a steady rate, which is vital given the episodic secretion of hormones. Only a tiny fraction of total circulating hormone is biologically active (0.1–5%) and this is the unbound portion. The important circulating binding proteins can be remembered by another feline mnemonic:

CATTS

C **C**orticosteroid-binding globulin (**C**BG)
A **A**lbumin
T **T**ranscalciferin (vitamin D transport globulin)
T **T**hyroxine-binding globulin (**T**BG)
S **S**ex-hormone-binding globulin (**S**HBG)

The endocrine organs

There are various endocrine organs located throughout the body with very different properties. Think of them anatomically from top to bottom:

- Hypothalamus
- Pituitary (anterior and posterior) gland
- Thyroid glands
- Parathyroid glands
- Adrenal glands
- Pancreas
- Placenta
- Ovaries
- Testes

Hypothalamus

Anatomy

APPS

Anterior hypothalamic area controls the **P**arasympathetic nervous system

Posterior hypothalamic area controls the **S**ympathetic nervous system

Anterior pituitary gland

Anatomy

The pituitary has been called the master gland of the body because of its central role in governing homeostasis, maintaining the reproductive cycle, and directing the activity of other glands. The pituitary is located in the sella turcica or in other words:

The **PIT SITS** in the Turkish saddle.

It is called a saddle because it has a floor and an anterior and posterior wall. The pituitary consists of two separate lobes, the anterior (adenohypophysis) and the posterior (neurohypophysis), and they are linked by an intermediate lobe which is vestigial in humans.

Histology

The bulk of the adenohypophysis is composed of epithelial cells flanked by vascular sinusoids. Three distinct cell types are seen among epithelial cells that are stained with dyes such as haematoxylin and eosin:

ABC

A **A**cidophils have cytoplasm that stains red or orange; somatotropes, lactotropes
B **B**asophils have cytoplasm that stains a bluish colour; gonadotropes, corticotropes, thyrotropes
C **C**hromophobes have cytoplasm that stains very poorly

TP FLAG – **T**he **P**ituitary **FLAG** – the master gland is so great it should have its own flag!

Anterior pituitary hormones	**Histology**
TSH	Thyrotropes
Prolactin	Lactotropes
FSH	Gonadotropes
LH	Gonadotropes
ACTH	Corticotropes
GH	Somatotropes

The hormones of the hypothalamus and the anterior pituitary gland

Hypothalamic releasing hormone	Effect on pituitary	Pituitary stimulating hormone	Hormone
TRH	+	TSH	Thyroid hormones T_4, T_3
Dopamine	–	Prolactin	
GnRH	+	FSH	Oestrogen or testosterone
LHRH	+		
GnRH	+	LH	Oestrogen or testosterone
LH-releasing hormone	+		
CRH	+	ACTH	Cortisol
GHRH	+	GH	IGF-1
Somatostatin	–		

An easy way to remember the hypothalamic hormones that have an inhibitory effect on anterior pituitary hormones is that they are **SAD**:

S   **S**omatostatin
A   **A**ntagonistic
D   **D**opamine

Also these are the only two hormones that do not have **releasing** in their names.

Hypopituitarism

Hypopituitarism can have an acute onset or be insidious and it may affect only one pituitary hormone, a few, or all of them. Panhypopituitarism of the anterior pituitary gland can be partial or complete and can be associated with diabetes insipidus in some cases. The extent of the dysfunction will determine the severity of the signs and symptoms. The causes of hypopituitarism are:

HIPO-PITS

H   **H**ypophysectomy
I   **I**rradiation of pituitary
P   **P**ituitary adenoma/**P**rolactinoma
O   **O**(a)uto-immune
P   **P**eri-pituitary glioma/cranio-**p**haryngioma
I   **I**nfection – meningitis/encephalitis
T   **T**rauma – skull fracture/surgery
S   **S**phenoid menigioma/**S**heehan's syndrome/**S**arcoidosis

Sheehan's syndrome

SHE HAS SHEehan's syndrome

The commonest vascular cause of panhypopituitarism is Sheehan's syndrome. It is exclusive to females. Post-partum pituitary necrosis leads to hypopituitarism. The first symptom is that lactation does not occur and the other symptoms of hypopituitarism follow. There is also a lack of menses. It is possible that prolonged shock in other situations may lead to panhypopituitarism.

Pituitary tumours

The most common cases of panhypopituitarism are pituitary or suprasellar tumours. They are usually benign and account for 10% of intracranial tumours. They lead to symptoms that are due to the pressure effects on the structures that surround the tumour, such as the optic chiasm and the hypothalamus. Common tumours include adenomas, prolactinomas and craniopharyngiomas.

Effects of pituitary or suprasellar tumours

HEAD AKE

H Headache, often severe in nature and persistent
E Eye – visual field defects (usually bitemporal hemianopia)
A Appetite may be disturbed leading to hyperphagia, thirst can also feature
D Diabetes insipidus
A Atrophy of optic area may be revealed by fundoscopy
K Korsakoff's-like syndrome with recent memory loss may occur due to pressure on the third ventricle
E Excess hormones may be secreted by tumours, ie prolactin by prolactinomas

Investigation of hypopituitarism

How People Investigate Hypopituitarism

H History – ie radiotherapy in the past
P Physical examination – assessment of visual fields
I Imaging – (X-rays, CT or MRI); lateral and antero-posterior radiographs of the skull may show an expanded pituitary fossa but this does not necessarily mean that a tumour is responsible for this; therefore, a CT or MRI scan is needed; angiography may be used if an aneurysm is suspected of impinging on the pituitary
H Hormone measurements (PRL, GH, TSH and gonadotrophins) can help diagnose the nature of a pituitary tumour but careful diagnosis is needed

Management of hypopituitarism

For hormone replacement therapy steroids should **ALWAYS** be given before thyroid hormones, remember that **s**teroids begin with an **S** and precede the **T** of **t**hyroid alphabetically. Other hormone replacement therapy then follows.

Isolated deficiencies of pituitary stimulating hormones

TSH disorders

Isolated TSH disorders are rare.

PRL (Prolactin)

PRL causes milk protein synthesis and excretion in breast tissue ducts and lobules and stimulates the growth of ducts and lobules.

Factors stimulating PRL secretion

SEEP ON

S **S**uckling an infant
E **E**xpecting, ie pregnant
E **E**xamining the breast which causes stress
P **P**uberty
O **O**estrogen and progesterone
N **N**ight-time

Clinical features of hyperprolactinaemia

COLD

C Menstrual **C**ycle is erratic leading to anovulatory **C**ycles or amenorrhoea
O **O**estrogen levels decreased leading to osteoporosis or cardiovascular disease
L **L**ibido is decreased
D **D**yspareunia can occur due to low oestrogen levels

Causes of hyperprolactinaemia

PIT

P   **P**regnancy is by far the most common cause
I   **I**atrogenic – ie taking **OCP**s that contain oestrogen
T   **T**umours of the pituitary

Prolactinomas

Pituitary tumours can be divided into two groups: those that affect the pituitary stalk and lead to dopamine deficiency and those that secrete PRL (prolactinomas). Prolactinomas are classified as microprolactinomas if they are less than 1 cm in diameter and macroprolactinomas if they are larger.

Clinical features of macroprolactinomas

GAIL PHD

G   **G**alactorrhoea
A   **A**menorrhoea
I   **I**mpotence in males
L   **L**ethargy
P   **P**ressure effects of the tumour in the head
H   Loss of secondary sexual **H**air
D   **D**epression

Gonadotrophin disorders

Isolated tumours of FSH and LH are rare.

ACTH disorders

Adreno**CORTI**cotrophic hormone (ACTH) is synthesised and secreted by **CORTI**cotrophic cells of the adrenal gland and stimulates **CORTI**sol.

Isolated ACTH deficiency

Is very rare.

Diagnosis of isolated ACTH deficiency

ACTH

A Low plasma **A**CTH levels
C Low plasma **C**ortisol levels
T Cortisol does not rise normally in response to short synacthen **T**est
H Cortisol does not rise normally in response to insulin **H**ypoglycaemia

ACTH excess

ACTH excess such as due to an ACTH-secreting adenoma leads to pituitary-dependent Cushing's syndrome.

GH disorders

↓ GH in child (before epiphyseal fusion)	**↑ GH in child (before epiphyseal fusion)**
Short stature	Gigantism
↓ GH in adult	**↑ GH in adult**
Clinically silent	Acromegaly

Acromegaly

A disease due to hypersecretion of GH from a pituitary tumour in adulthood. Usually presents between the ages of 30 and 50.

Signs

Draw a caricature, and exaggerate the features to enhance your recall of them.

- **The head and neck**

  - Prominent supraorbital ridge (frontal bossing)
  - Visual field defects such as bitemporal quadrantanopia progresses to bitemporal hemianopia; local mass effects of a pituitary tumour
  - Broad bridge of the nose
  - Prominent nasolabial folds
  - Thick lips
  - Interdental separation
  - Large tongue
  - Acne
  - Prognathism (prominent jaw)
  - Husky voice, due to thickening of the vocal cords
  - Multinodular goitre

- **The trunk**

  - Heart failure
  - Hypertension
  - Galactorrhoea (spontaneous milk production)
  - Enlarged viscera: liver/spleen

- **The limbs**

  - Proximal myopathy
  - Premature osteoarthritis
  - Spade-like hands and feet
  - Thick greasy skin
  - Tightening of rings on fingers
  - Carpal tunnel syndrome
  - Peripheral oedema

Complications

ABCDEFGH

A **A**cromegaly
B **B**lood pressure increases/large **B**owel tumours (benign or malignant)
C **C**ardiomyopathy/**C**arpal tunnel syndrome
D **D**iabetes mellitus
E **E**nlarged viscera
F **F**ield defects
G **G**alactorrhoea
H **H**eart failure/**H**ypertension

Investigations

GO MASSIVE

G **G**rowth hormone measurement in isolation, variable and therefore random measurements are not diagnostic
O **O**GTT with GH measurement; the definitive test for acromegaly
M **M**RI or CT scan of pituitary fossa
A Visual **A**cuity
S **S**kin thickness
S **S**ee old photos and compare with new for changes in facial features
I Serum **I**GF-1, a reliable measure of GH secretion over previous 24 hours
V **V**isual fields
E **E**CG

Treatment

TEDS

T **T**rans-sphenoidal surgery is the gold standard
E **E**xternal irradiation, this is for older patients or if surgery is not possible
D **D**opamine agonists – bromocriptine, cabergoline
S **S**omatostatin analogues – octreotide, lanreotide

Posterior pituitary gland

Anatomy

The posterior pituitary is nervous tissue and this is reflected in the name ***neuro****hypophysis*.

Histology

The neurohypophysis consists of the terminals of axons extending down from cell bodies in the hypothalamus. It also contains numerous glia cells ('pituicytes').

The hormones of the posterior pituitary

OA

O **O**xytocin
A **A**DH (or vasopressin)

ADH

Not enough ADH = diabetes insipidus, **CAN'T HOLD ON TO THEIR WATER**

Too much ADH = SIADH, **CAN'T GET RID OF THEIR WATER**

Diabetes insipidus

Symptoms

TDP; To **D**o **P**ee

T **T**hirst
D **D**ilute urine
P **P**olyuria (some pass more than 10 litres a day)

Causes of cranial DI

DI SUMMIT

D **DIDMOAD** (familial syndrome of **DI**, **DM**, **o**ptic **a**trophy and **d**eafness)
I **I**nherited (autosomal dominant)
S **S**arcoidosis
U **U**nknown in 33% of cases
M **M**etastases
M **M**eningitis
I **I**njury to head
T **T**umour of pituitary

Causes of nephrogenic DI

CHILD PP (as in child peepee)

C   **C**alcium is high
H   **H**ydronephrosis
I   **I**nherited
L   **L**ow potassium
D   **D**rugs (lithium)
P   **P**yelonephritis
P   **P**regnancy

Interpreting the water deprivation test

After a desmopressin injection:

Concentrated urine = **C**onfirmation of true DI.

Desmopressin is also used in the management of DI.

SIADH

Causes

SIADH

S   **S**urgery – 24–48 h afterwards
I   **I**diopathic/**I**ntracranial: infection, head injury, CVA
A   **A**cute and chronic pulmonary disease
D   **D**eficiency of cortisol/**D**rugs: opiates, antiepileptics, cytotoxics, anti-psychotics
H   **H**ypothyroidism/**H**yponatraemia

Clinical features

CCF (**C**an't **C**lear **F**luids)

C   **C**onfusion
C   **C**oma
F   **F**its

Thyroid gland

Anatomy

An adult's **T**hyroid gland is **T**wenty grams and lies in front of the **T**hyroid cartilage, close to the first part of the **T**rachea. It has **T**wo lobes, connected by an isthmus. It **T**ravels with the **T**hyroid cartilage on swallowing.

Histology

The thyroid gland is composed of hollow sacs called thyroid follicles which are lined by a layer of cuboidal epithelium and contain a colloid. Lobules consist of 20–40 follicles with a common blood supply.

The thyroid gland contains most of the body's total iodine which is converted into T_4 (thyroxine) and T_3 (triiodothyronine). There is **more T_4** than T_3. Four is a bigger number than three, so remember there is more of it. T_4 can be regarded as a pro-hormone and it is converted into a biologically active form, T_3. Most of the circulating T_3 and T_4 is bound and inactive. **Remember that bound prisoners are not free to act.** When T_3 is unbound it is active.

C cells

Parafollicular cells (**C** cells) lie next to the follicles and secrete the hormone **C**alcitonin which lowers **C**alcium.

Actions of T_3/T_4

THYROID

T   Increases body **T**emperature
H   **H**eart – promotes normal cardiac function
Y   Increases lipol**Y**sis
R   **R**eproductive – promotes normal female reproductive ability and lactation
O   **O**rganogenesis – promotes normal neuronal development in the fetus and infant and promotes normal neuronal function in adults
I   **I**ncreases appetite/**I**ncreases basal metabolic rate
D   Promotes normal function and **D**evelopment of muscles

Hypothyroidism

Endemic cretinism is a severe neurological disorder occurring in areas of **endemic** goitre in **children** who have goitrous and iodine-deficient mothers.

Symptoms of hypothyroidism

MOM'S SO TIRED

Hypothyroidism is 10 times more common in females than males and occurs mainly in middle life.

M **M**emory loss
O **O**besity
M **M**alar flush/**M**enorrhagia
S **S**lowness
S **S**kin and hair become dry
O **O**nset is gradual
T **T**ired
I **I**ntolerance to cold
R **R**aised blood pressure
E **E**nergy levels are low
D **D**epressed

Signs

Draw a caricature, and exaggerate the features to enhance your recall of them.

- **The head and neck**

  - Psychological changes: depression, dementia, mental slowness, psychosis
  - Lethargy
  - Cerebellar ataxia
  - Hair loss on scalp
  - Eyebrow, loss of lateral one-third
  - Palar conjunctiva and anaemia
  - Toad face
  - Dry skin/hair
  - Large tongue
  - Excess clothing due to cold intolerance
  - Corneal arcus
  - Xanthelasma
  - Goitre and hoarse voice

- **The trunk**

  - Pericardial/pleural effusions
  - Ascites
  - Cardiac dilatation
  - Hypothermia
  - Weight gain
  - Hypertension
  - Constipation
  - Bradycardia

- **The limbs**

  - Carpal tunnel syndrome
  - Cold peripheries
  - Tendon xanthomata
  - Non-pitting oedema of eyelids and hands
  - Slow relaxing reflexes
  - Myalgia
  - Muscular hypertrophy

Treatment

2Ts

Thyroid hormone replacement with **T**$_4$.

Monitor **T**SH levels.

Hyperthyroidism

Symptoms

SWEATING

S	**S**weating
W	**W**eight loss
E	**E**motional lability
A	**A**ppetite is increased
T	**T**remor/**T**achycardia due to AF
I	**I**ntolerance to heat/**I**rregular menstruation/**I**rritability
N	**N**ervousness
G	**G**oitre and **G**astrointestinal problems (loose stools/diarrhoea)

Signs of hyperthyroidism

Draw a caricature, and exaggerate the features to enhance your recall of them.

- **The head and neck**

  - Psychological changes such as irritability, emotional lability, psychosis
  - Hair loss
  - Sweating
  - Lid lag
  - Decreased weight
  - Increased appetite
  - Heat intolerance
  - Goitre
  - Pruritis

- **The trunk**

  - Tachycardia
  - Gynaecomastia
  - Diarrhoea
  - Oligomenorrhoea
  - Infertility

- **The limbs**

  - Palmar erythema
  - Fine tremor
  - Warm peripheries
  - Sweaty palms

Other hormones involved in thyrotoxicosis

Can't **S**ettle

- **C** **C**atecholamines, many of the features of thyrotoxicosis are due to increased sensitivity to circulating catecholamines such as adrenaline
- **S** **S**HBG is found in increased levels in thyrotoxic patients with gynaecomastia and infertility

Grave's disease

Also known as Grave's ophthalmopathy, thyroid-associated ophthalmopathy, dysthyroid eye disease and infiltrative eye disease. In **G**rave's disease, the thyroid-stimulating auto-immunoglobulins are of the Ig**G** class.

Signs of Grave's disease

Draw a caricature, and exaggerate the features to enhance your recall of them.

- **The head and neck**

  - Exophthalmos
  - Lid retraction
  - Lid lag
  - Periorbital puffiness
  - Grittiness in eyes
  - Increased lacrimation
  - Chemosis
  - Conjunctival oedema and ulceration
  - Swelling
  - Redness
  - Proptosis
  - Ophthalmoplegia, photophobia, blurred vision, diplopia
  - Visual failure due to optic nerve compression by the extraocular muscles
  - Papilloedema is a sign of a dangerous rise in ocular and orbital pressure
  - Diffuse goitre with bruit

- **The trunk**

  - Tachycardia with bounding pulse
  - Weight loss
  - Vitiligo

- **The limbs**

  - Fine tremor of hands
  - Slow relaxing reflexes
  - Proximal myopathy
  - Pretibial myxoedema over anterolateral aspect of lower legs
  - Thyroid acropachy (like clubbing) and periosteal reaction in the bones of the forearm

Management of Hyper-thyroidism

BART

B **B**eta blockers, such as propranolol
A **A**nti-thyroid drugs, such as carbimazole
R **R**adio-iodine treatment
T **T**hyroidectomy

Thyroid cancers

Thyroid cancers

P FMA (Most common to least common)

Papillary
Follicular   Prognosis worsens
Medullary   down the order
Anaplastic

Clinical features of thyroid cancers

CHIEF

C **C**hange in voice
H **H**ard mass
I **I**ncreased lymph node size
E **E**nlargement is rapid
F **F**ixed mass

Parathyroid glands

Hypoparathyroidism is associated with **hypo**calcaemia; **hyper**parathyroidism is associated with **hyper**calcaemia.

Clinical features of primary hyperparathyroidism

Bones   Bone pain
Stones Kidney stones
Groans Abdominal pain
Moans   Emotional upset: depression, anxiety

Adrenal glands

Anatomy

The **medulla** is in the **middle** of the adrenal gland and the **cortex** is the **covering**.

The blood supply flows from the **c**ortex to the **m**edulla, in alphabetical order – **C** precedes **M**.

The adrenal cortex has four layers and secretes steroid hormones

Glasses **F**eel **R**ight, **M**ake **G**ood **S**ight

Coronal section starting externally: first there is the capsule and then the zona layers and their respective steroid hormones:

Layers of the cortex	Steroid hormones produced	Specific examples of hormones
Zona **G**lomerulosa	**M**ineralocorticoids	Aldosterone
Zona **F**asciculata	**G**lucocorticoids	Cortisol
Zona **R**eticulata	**S**ex hormones	DHEA and other weak androgens

Alternatively for layers:

GFR (**G**lomerular **F**iltration **R**ate, convenient since adrenal glands sit above the kidneys).

Mineralocorticoids

Aldosterone is a miner**AL**ocorticoid. (Ignore the CORTI in mineralocorticoid, remember that the **AL** comes first.) Aldosterone acts on intranuclear mineralocorticoid receptors in the distal renal tubule to promote sodium moving **into** cells and potassium moving **out**:

Sod**IN**um, P**OUT**assium.

Glucocorticoids

CORTIsol is a gluco**CORTI**coid.

Actions of glucocorticoids

CORTI

C **C**atabolic actions on muscles
O **O**ther hormone effects are modified
R **R**epair processes and collagen synthesis in bone and soft tissues are inhibited
T **T**hey facilitate requirements of daytime activity and are needed for the stress response
I **I**nfluence glucose homeostasis

Adrenal androgens

Relatively unimportant post utero.

Adrenal medulla

Releases adrenaline (epinephrine) after which the adrenal glands are named.

Disorders of the adrenal cortex

Adrenocortical insufficiency

Definition

Deficiency of **MAG**

M **M**ineralocorticoids
A **A**ndrogens
G **G**lucocorticoids

Or alternatively of **MGS** from the mnemonic '**G**lasses **F**eel **R**ight, **M**akes **G**ood **S**ight'

Addison's disease

Addison's is in**Ad**equate **Ad**renocorticoids.

Or **Ad**renocorticoids do not **ADD UP**

Causes of Addison's disease

ADDISON

A **A**utoimmune (90% cases)
D **D**egenerative (amyloid)
D **D**rugs (ketoconazole)
I **I**nfections (TB, HIV)
S **S**econdary (low ACTH); hypopituitarism
O **O**thers – adrenal bleeding
N **N**eoplasia (secondary carcinoma)

Signs of Addison's disease

Draw a caricature, and exaggerate the features to enhance your recall of them.

● **The head and neck**

■ Hair loss from scalp and axilla
■ Vitiligo
■ Increased skin pigmentation

Clinical presentation of Addisonian crisis

THE A D CRISIS

T **T**achycardia
H **H**ypotension
E **E**yes are sunken
A **A**bdominal pain and **A**norexia
D **D**izziness especially postural/**D**ehydrated
C **C**ramps
R **R**igid abdomen
I **I**ncreased calcium
S **S**erum **S**odium is low
I **I**ll patient with a fever who is vomiting
S **S**kin turgor is lost

Management of Addison's disease

Hydro**CORTI**sone, fluids and electrolytes

The short synacthen test

SYNACTH

An initial blood sample is taken to assess the baseline level of cortisol. An injection to stimulate the body's production of cortisol is given. A blood sample is taken at 30 min and 60 min after the stimulation to measure the cortisol level.

S **S**timulation test for primary adrenal insufficiency
Y **Y** not try the long synacthen test or a depot synacthen test if secondary adrenal insufficiency
N **N**o rise in serum cortisol in response to synacthen in hypoadrenal patients
A Used to **A**scertain that the **A**drenals are functioning normally after a prolonged course of corticosteroids
C **C**hecks the amount of **C**ortisol in the body
T Synacthen is **T**etracosactrin, the first 24 amino acids of ACTH
H Used in the diagnosis of **H**ypoadrenalism

Cushing's syndrome

CUSHing's is where **C**ortisol is **GUSH**ing

Cushing's syndrome

Chronic glucocorticoid excess of which 90% are ACTH-dependent and 10% are ACTH-independent. Causes of Cushing's syndrome include Cushing's disease and iatrogenic causes such as steroids.

Cushing's disease

ACTH-dependent pituitary adenoma.

Cushing's **S**yndrome is the **SUM** of all causes whereas Cushing's **D**isease is ACTH-**D**ependent.

Signs of Cushing's syndrome

Draw a caricature, and exaggerate the features to enhance your recall of them.

- **The head and neck**

  - Frontal balding
  - Moon face
  - Acne
  - Plethoric complexion
  - Hirsutism

- **The trunk**

  - Kyphosis
  - Buffalo hump (fat pad)
  - Gynaecomastia in males
  - Central obesity (due to altered fat distribution)
  - Purple striae on abdomen, breasts, thighs
  - Pigmentation in ACTH-dependent cases, in areas exposed to sunlight
  - Thin skin
  - Hair growth on forearms in particular
  - Tissue wasting
  - Predisposition to infection
  - Bad wound healing

- **The limbs**

  - Proximal myopathy
  - Pathological fractures
  - Ankle oedema (salt and water retention due to excess cortisol)

Investigation of Cushing's syndrome

OTFC; **O**ur **T**ests **F**or **C**ushing's

O **O**vernight dexamethasone suppression test
T **T**wenty-four-hour urinary free cortisol (an alternative)
F **F**orty-eight-hour dexamethasone suppression test
C **C**ircadian rhythm of cortisol secretion

Management of Cushing's syndrome

RAPID

R **R**adiotherapy of the pituitary
A **A**drenal surgery for an adrenal adenoma or carcinoma
P **P**ituitary surgery, gold standard for Cushing's disease via transsphenoidal route
I **I**atrogenic causes must have the medication stopped
D **D**rug therapy, ketoconazole to reduce plasma cortisol

Disorders of aldosterone secretion

Clinical features of hypoaldosteronism

PASH

P **P**otassium is high
A **A**ldosterone resistance
S **S**odium depletion
H **H**ypotension

Clinical presentation of primary hyperaldosteronism (Conn's syndrome)

HARPS

H **H**ypertension
A **A**ldosterone is raised
R **R**enin is lowered
P **P**otassium is decreased
S **S**odium raised

Investigations of hyperaldosteronism

ABCD

A **A**drenal scintigraphy: allows distinction between Conn's syndrome and bilateral adrenal hyperplasia by measuring adrenal vein aldosterone levels
B **B**loods (obviously do this first). Plasma aldosterone will be raised
C **C**T/MRI, visualises the adrenals
D **D**iurnal and postural measurements of aldosterone and renin

Causes of secondary hyperaldosteronism

CLAN

C **C**ongestive cardiac failure
L **L**iver cirrhosis
A **A**ccelerated hypertension
N **N**ephrotic syndrome

Disorders of the adrenal medulla

Phaeochromocytoma

Clinical features of phaeochromocytoma

PHAE

P **P**alpitations, flushing and nervousness
H **H**ypertension
A **A**ttacks of headache
E **E**pisodic sweating (diaphoresis)

Epidemiology of phaeochromocytoma

10% COME

C 10% in **C**hildren
O 10% **O**ccur in families
M 10% are **M**alignant
E 10% are **E**xtra-adrenal

This is also a good way to remember that phaeo**CHROM**ocytoma affects the **CHROM**affin cells of the adrenal medulla, as **CHRO-ME**.

Management of phaeochromocytoma

ABC

A **A**lpha blockers
B **B**eta blockers
C **C**urgery

Multiple endocrine neoplasia (MEN)

Types of **MEN**

There are **three** types of **MEN** (1, 2a, 2b) and **three** letters in the word **men**.

Pancreas

Anatomy and histology

The pancreas has endocrine and exocrine actions. The exocrine cells are arranged in sac-like glands with ducts called acini. These cells produce enzymes for the digestive system.

The endocrine units are called the islets of Langerhans and they are scattered throughout the pancreas.

Endocrine secretions

BAD

B   **B**eta cells secrete insulin
A   **A**lpha cells secrete glucagon
D   **D** cells secrete somatostatin

Exocrine secretions

TALC

T   **T**rypsin, breaks down proteins
A   **A**mylase, breaks down starches
L   **L**ipase, breaks down fats
C   **C**hymotrypsin, breaks down proteins

Action of insulin

INsul**IN** stimulates **2** things to go **IN 2** cells: potassium and glucose

Action of glucagon

Gluca has **Gone** to **cAMP** to bring **out Glucose**: glucagon elevates glucose by cAMP involvement

Diabetes mellitus type I

Signs and symptoms of acute presentation

Draw a caricature, and exaggerate the features to enhance your recall of them.

- **Diabetic ketoacidosis (DKA)**

  - Coma
  - Confusion
  - Drowsiness
  - Nausea/vomiting
  - Polyuria
  - Polydipsia
  - Signs of dehydration (dry mucous membranes, decreased tissue turgor)
  - Ketotic breath
  - Kussmaul breathing (deep and rapid)
  - Abdominal pain

- **Hypoglycaemia**

  - Coma
  - Focal neurological symptoms
  - Personality change
  - Fitting
  - Confusion
  - Dizziness
  - Hunger
  - Pallor
  - Sweating
  - Tremor
  - Tachycardia
  - Palpitations

Clinical features of DKA

DKA

D **D**ehydrated/**D**rowsiness that can lead to coma
K **K**etoacidosis/**K**ussmaul breathing/**K**+(potassium) drops
A **A**cetone breath/**A**cidosis/**A**bdominal pain

Causes of DKA

5 Is

I **I**nfection (UTI, pneumonia)
I **I**schaemia (cardiac, mesenteric)
I **I**nfarction (MI)
I **I**gnorance (poor control)
I **I**ntoxication (alcohol)

Management of DKA

PANICS

P **P**otassium
A **A**cidosis: if pH <7.30 get urgent advice
N **N**ormal saline
I **I**nsulin infusion
C **C**atheter and **C**ultures (urine and blood)
S **S**tomach aspiration/**S**ubcutaneous heparin

Clinical features of hypoglycaemia

5Ss and 2Cs

Starving (feel hungry)
Shaky (tremors)
Sweating
Sky-high pulse (tachycardia)
Sleepy or irritable

Later:

Convulsions
Coma

Causes of hypoglycaemia

EXPLAIN

EX **EX**ogenous drugs (insulin, oral hypoglycaemics, alcohol, pentamidine, quinine, quinolones)
P **P**ituitary insufficiency (no GH or cortisol)
L **L**iver failure (no glycogen stores)
A **A**drenal failure (no cortisol)
I **I**nsulinomas/**I**mmune hypoglycaemia
N **N**on-pancreatic neoplasms (retroperitoneal fibrosarcoma)

Signs and symptoms of diabetes mellitus type II

Draw a caricature, and exaggerate the features to enhance your recall of them.

- **General**

  - Polyuria
  - Polydipsia
  - Lethargy
  - Infections (eg candidiasis)

- **Diabetic skin**

  - Necrobiosis lipoidica diabeticorum
  - Granuloma annulare
  - Diabetic dermopathy

- **Diabetic feet**

  - Ischaemia
  - Neuropathy
  - Dry skin
  - Reduced subcutaneous tissue
  - Corns and calluses
  - Ulcers
  - Gangrene
  - Charcot's arthropathy
  - Signs of peripheral neuropathy
  - Decreased foot pulses

Complications of diabetes mellitus

KEVINS

K   **K**idney; Nephropathy
E   **E**ye disease; retinopathy and cataracts
V   **V**ascular; coronary artery disease, cerebrovascular disease, peripheral vascular disease
I   **I**nfective; TB, recurrent UTIs
N   **N**euromuscular; Peripheral neuropathy
S   **S**kin; Necrobiosis lipoidica diabeticorum, granuloma annulare, diabetic dermopathy

Management of diabetes mellitus

ABCDEFGH

A **A**dvice: diet, exercise, smoking cessation, weight control
B **B**lood pressure management, target is <130/80 mmHg
C **C**holesterol management, ideally less then 5 mmol/l
D **D**iabetes management, blood glucose within 4–7 mmol/l
     (diet control firstly if Type II then oral hypoglycaemics +/–
     insulin. Type I diabetics have a total insulin requirement)
E **E**ye checks
F **F**eet checks
G **G**uardian drugs: aspirin to prevent heart problems, ACE
     inhibitors to prevent heart disease, stroke, kidney disease
     and eye disease
H **H**bA1c < 7%: indicator of glycaemic control over past two
     months

The testes

Anatomy and histology

The testis is composed of coiled **S**eminiferou**S** tubules where
Spermatogene**S**i**S** occurs, resulting in the production of **S**perm.
Between the tubules are in**T**ers**T**i**T**ial cells which produce
Tes**T**os**T**erone. The stimulation after puberty comes from the
pituitary hormones FSH and LH.

The testes in infancy

Shortly after the infant leaves his mother's abdomen his testes
leave his abdomen and descend to the scrotum.

The testes in puberty

In the male, puberty is initiated by the pulsatile nocturnal
secretion of LH. **L**H acts on **L**eydig cells (interstitial cells) to
promote steroid production. F**S**H acts on **S**ertoli cells to regulate
Spermatogenesis.

The sequence of development of secondary sexual characteristics in the male

Go **B**oy **G**o

G   **G**enital development
B   **B**ody hair growth increases (pubic and axillary)
G   **G**rowth spurt, muscles and bones develop

Impotence

Some causes of impotence

IMPOTENCES

I   **I**liac arteriosclerosis
M   **M**icropenis
P   **P**eyronie's disease
O   **O**rgan failure, heart failure
T   **T**hyrotoxicosis/**T**oo much glucose; DM
E   **E**motional factors
N   **N**europathy of autonomic system
C   **C**ushing's syndrome
E   **E**thanol (alcoholism)
S   **S**moking

Klinefelter's syndrome

Signs and symptoms

Draw a caricature, and exaggerate the features to enhance your recall of them.

● **The head and neck**

■ Mild learning difficulties in childhood
■ Slow verbal development
■ Clumsiness
■ Tall stature (with long legs, arm span is greater than height)
■ High-pitched voice

● **The trunk**

■ Obesity
■ Gynaecomastia
■ Small, firm pea-like testes
■ Small penis
■ Secondary sexual hair is sparse and with a female distribution

The ovaries

Anatomy and histology

Each female is born with approximately half a million ovarian follicles and when they are finished, menopause ensues.

The sequence of development of secondary sexual characteristics in the female

TAG Me

T	**T**helarche (development of breasts) 9–11 years
A	**A**drenarche (development of pubic hair) 12–13 years
G	**G**rowth spurt 12–14 years
Me	**Me**narche (commence menses) 13–15 years

Menstrual cycle disorder

Amenorrhoea	=	**A**bsent periods
Oligomenorrhoea	=	**O**ccasional periods
Primary amenorrhoea	=	At **P**uberty
Secondary amenorrhoea	=	**S**ubsequent to puberty

Signs and symptoms of Turner's syndrome

Draw a caricature, and exaggerate the features to enhance your recall of them.

- **The head and neck**
  - Short stature
  - Low hairline
  - High-arched palate
  - Night sweats
  - Hot flushes
  - Deafness
  - Short webbed neck

- **The trunk**

  - Thin skin
  - Decreased axillary or pubic hair
  - Widely spaced nipples
  - Shield chest
  - Signs of coarctation of aorta
  - Vertebral dysplasia
  - Multiple naevi
  - Vaginal dryness
  - Dyspareunia

- **The limbs**

  - Increased carrying angles of arm (cubitus valgus)
  - Short metacarpals (especially 4th)
  - Hypoplastic nails
  - Lymphoedema

Polycystic ovary syndrome (PCOS)

Clinical presentation

PCOS PAL

P	**P**olycystic ovaries on ultrasound
C	**C**ycles are erratic or amenorrhoea
O	**O**besity and hirsutism
S	**S**ubfertility
P	**P**rolactin elevated mildly
A	**A**ndrogens elevated modestly
L	**L**H elevated significantly

Signs and symptoms

Draw a caricature, and exaggerate the features to enhance your recall of them.

- **The head and neck**

  - Alopecia – male pattern balding
  - Hirsutism
  - Acne

- **The trunk**
  - Obesity
  - Hypertension
  - Acanthosis nigricans: thickening and hyperpigmentation of the skin of the axillae, neck and intertriginous areas
  - Menstrual irregularities (oligo- or amenorrhoea)

Disorders of male secondary sexual differentiation

Gynaecomastia

Causes of gynaecomastia

GYNAECOMASTIA

G **G**enetic disorder (Klinefelter's)
Y **Y**oung boy (pubertal)*
N **N**eonate*
A **A**lcoholism
E O**E**strogen
C **C**irrhosis/**C**imetidine/**C**alcium **C**hannel blockers
O **O**ld age*
M **M**arijuana
S **S**pironolactone
T **T**umours (**T**esticular and adrenal)
I **I**soniazid/**I**nhibition of testosterone
A **A**ntifungal (ketoconazole)

*Asterisk indicates physiological cause.

Disorders of female secondary sexual differentiation

Hirsutism

Treatment of hirsutism

PACT

P **P**sychological support
A **A**nti-androgens – spironolactone, finasteride
C **C**osmetic treatments – wax creams, electrolysis, shaving
T **T**umour that is the cause of virilisation should be excluded

Hirsutism versus virilism

> **H**irsutism: **H**air on body like a male
> **V**irilism: **V**oice and rest of secondary sexual characteristics like a male.

Virilisation

Clinical presentation of virilisation

SHAVED

S   **S**erum testosterone is raised
H   **H**irsutism
A   **A** typical male pattern frontal balding is seen
V   **V**oice deepens
E   **E**nlargement of the clitoris
D   **D**evelopment of male pattern muscle

Side-effects of steroids

MS. CUSHINGS

M   **M**yopathy/'**M**oon' face
S   p**S**ychiatric symptoms; depression

C   **C**ataracts
U   **U**p all night (sleep disturbances)
S   **S**uppression of HPA axis/**S**pots (acne)
H   **H**ypertension/buffalo **H**ump
I   **I**nfections
N   **N**ecrosis (avascular)
G   **G**ain weight/**G**lucose increased; DM
S   **S**triae/**S**limming of bones ie osteoporosis

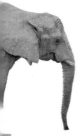

6. Gastroenterology

Anatomy

Diaphragm apertures

Spinal levels

- 'Vena cava' (inferior) = **8** letters = T**8**
- 'Oesophagus' = **10** letters = T**10**
- 'Aortic hiatus' = **12** letters = T**12**

Contents

3 holes, each with **3** things going through it

- Aortic hiatus: aorta, thoracic duct, azygous vein
- Oesophageal hiatus: oesophagus, vagal trunks, left gastric vessels
- Caval foramen: inferior vena cava (IVC), right phrenic nerve, lymph nodes

Clinical conditions

Constipation

Causes

DR. DOFEN

D **D**iet – poor, lacking fibre
R ano**R**ectal disease – anal fissure, anal stricture, rectal prolapse
D **D**rugs – opiates, anticholinergics, iron
O **O**bstruction of intestines – due to colorectal carcinoma, IBD, pelvic mass eg fetus, fibroids
F **F**luid intake restricted (dehydrated)
E **E**ndocrine – hypothyroid
N **N**euromuscular – spinal or pelvic nerve injury, aganglionosis, systemic sclerosis

Diarrhoea

Causes

DIOREA

D **D**rugs – antibiotics, PPIs, cimetidine, propranolol, cytotoxics, NSAIDs, digoxin, alcohol, laxative abuse
I **I**BD (Crohn's/UC)/**I**rritable bowel syndrome
O **O**vergrowth of bacteria
R Colo**R**ectal carcinoma
E Gastro**E**nteritis – viral, bacterial, parasites/protozoa/**E**ndocrine – thyrotoxicosis, Addison's disease
A **A**llergy to food

Dysphagia

Common causes

ABCD

Achalasia
Barrett's oesophagus/**B**enign oesophageal stricture from GORD
Carcinoma of oesophagus
Diffuse oesophageal spasm

Achalasia

One possible cause and one possible treatment

aCHAlasia

One possible cause = **CHA**gas disease

One possible treatment = calcium **CHA**nnel blockers

Barrett's oesophagus

Features

BARRett's

B **B**ecomes
A **A**denocarcinoma
R **R**esults from
R **R**eflux

Peptic ulcer

Risk factors

SHAZAN

S **S**moking/**S**picy foods
H *H. pylori*/**H**ypercalcaemia
A **A**spirin/**A**lcohol
Z **Z**ollinger–Ellison Syndrome
A **A**cidity
N **N**SAID use

Complications

HOP

H **H**aemorrhage
O **O**bstruction
P **P**erforation/**P**ain

Helicobacter pylori treatment regime

Triple therapy (for 7 days)

PAC

P   **P**PI, eg lansoprazole
A   **A**moxicillin
C   **C**larithromycin

If this fails, try quadruple therapy

To **M**ake **P**eptic ulcers **B**etter

T   **T**etracycline
M   **M**etronidazole
P   **P**PI
B   **B**ismuth

Abdomen distension

Causes

6 Fs

F   **F**at
F   **F**etus
F   **F**latus
F   **F**aeces
F   **F**luid
F   **F**lipping great tumour

Ascites

Common causes

4 Cs

Cirrhosis
Carcinomatosis
Cardiac failure
Cidney – nephrotic syndrome

Liver failure

Causes

HALTED

H Hepatitis – viral (Hep A,B,D,E)
A Autoimmune hepatitis
L Leptospirosis (infection)
T Toxins – *Amanita phalloides* mushrooms
E Enzyme deficiency – α_1-antitrypsin deficiency
D Drugs – paracetamol overdose, halothane, isoniazid

Cirrhosis

Causes

DR. HEPATICA

DR DRugs – amiodarone, methyldopa, methotrexate
H Hepatitis – viral hepatitis B,C
E Enzyme deficiency – α_1-antitrypsin deficiency
P Primary biliary cirrhosis/**P**rimary sclerosing cholangitis
A Alcohol abuse – chronic
T Tyrosinosis
I Indian childhood (galactosaemia)
C Cryptogenic – in 5–10%/**C**ystic fibrosis/**C**opper deposition; Wilson's disease/haemo-**C**hromatosis
A Autoimmune hepatitis

Chronic liver disease

Signs

ABCDEFGHIJ

A Asterixis ('liver flap')/**A**scites/**A**nkle oedema/**A**trophy of testicles
B Bruising/**B**P↓
C Clubbing/**C**olour change of nails; white (leuconychia)
D Dupuytren's contracture
E Erythema (palmar)/**E**ncephalopathy
F hepatic **F**oetor
G Gynaecomastia
H Hepato splenomegaly
I Increase in size of parotids
J Jaundice

Hepatocellular carcinoma

Causes

ABCD

A **A**flatoxins
B Hepatitis **B**
C **C**irrhosis/hepatitis **C**
D **D**rugs – anabolic steroids and contraceptives

Features

ABC

A **A**lphafeto protein ↑
B Vitamin **B$_{12}$**-binding protein (fibrolamellar – hepatocellular carcinoma)
C **C**alcium ↑ (biochemical evidence of paraneoplastic syndromes)

Inflammatory bowel disease (IBD)

Ulcerative colitis

Features

ULCERS IN Abdomen

U **U**lcers (mucosal and submucosal)
L **L**arge intestine (rectum always involved. May extend proximally to involve entire colon)
C **C**lubbing
E **E**xtra-intestinal manifestations
R **R**emnants of old ulcers (pseudopolyps)
S **S**tools bloody
I **I**nflamed, red, granular mucosa and sub mucosa
N **N**eutrophil invasion
A **A**bscesses in crypts

Definition of a severe attack

EAT STEroid

E **E**SR > 30 mm/h
A **A**lbumin < 30 g/l
T **T**emperature at 6 a.m. > 37.8°C
S **S**tool frequency > six stools/day with blood
T **T**achycardia > 90 beats/min
E **E**naemia – Haemoglobin (Hb) <10.5 g/dl

Complications

How **T**o **P**erform **GI C**olonoscopy

H **H**aemorrhage
T **T**oxic megacolon
P **P**erforation
G **G**allstones
C **C**olorectal carcinoma (in those with extensive disease for > 10 years)

Crohn's disease

Morphology and symptoms

CHRIS Has **T**oo **M**uch **D**iarrhoea and **A**bdominal pain

C **C**obblestone appearance of mucosa
H **H**igh temperature
R **R**educed lumen/**R**ose-thorn ulcers
I **I**ntestinal fistulae/**I**leo-caecal region commonly involved (40% of cases)
S **S**kip lesions
H **H**yperplasia of mesenteric lymph nodes
T **T**ransmural inflammation (all layers, may ulcerate)
M **M**alabsorption
D **D**iarrhoea (watery)
A **A**bdominal pain

Extraintestinal manifestations of IBD

A PIE SAC

A **A**phthous ulcers (Crohn's only)
P **P**yoderma gangrenosum
I **I** (eye) – iritis, uveitis, episcleritis, conjunctivitis
E **E**rythema nodosum
S **S**clerosing cholangitis
A **A**rthritis
C **C**lubbing

Management

SCAM

S **S**ulphasalazine
C **C**orticosteroids/**C**iprofloxacin
A **A**zathioprine
M **M**etronidazole/**M**ethotrexate

Indications for surgery

CHOP IT

C **C**arcinoma/**C**onnections abnormal ie fistulae
H **H**aemorrhage
O **O**bstruction
P **P**erforation
I **I**nfection
T failure to **T**hrive in children (Crohn's)

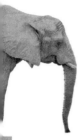

7. Haematology

Microcytic anaemia

Definition

Anaemia associated with low **MC**V (<80 fl) (**MiC**ro = ↓).

Causes

Females **S**uffer **T**his **C**ondition

This is commonly seen in up to 14% of menstruating women.

F   **Fe** (iron) deficiency (commonest cause)
S   **S**ideroblastic anaemia
T   **T**halassaemia
C   **C**hronic disease (often normocytic but may be microcytic)

Symptoms

Ltd

L   **L**ethargy
t   **t**iredness
d   **d**yspnoea

Signs

PIGSTY

P **P**allor of skin and mucous membranes
I **I**nflammation of lips; cheilitis (angular stomatitis)
G **G**lossitis: atrophy of tongue papillae
S **S**poon-shaped nails; koilonychia (in long-standing and severe cases)
T **T**achycardia (uncommon)
Y S**Y**stolic flow murmurs (uncommon)

Macrocytic anaemia

Definition

Anaemia associated with a high **MC**V (> 100 fl) (**MaC**ro = ↑).

Causes

Non-megaloblastic causes (ie non-B_{12} or folate deficiency causes):

On the hiking trip I **HELD** the **MAP**

H **H**aemolysis
E **E**ndocrine (hypothyroidism)
L **L**iver disease
D **D**rugs, eg hydroxyurea, azathioprine
M **M**yelodysplasia
A **A**lcohol excess
P **P**regnancy

As megaloblastic anaemia is a result of a vitamin B_{12} deficiency, which leads to pernicious anaemia (inability to absorb vitamin B_{12}), the features of both these conditions should be known:

Pernicious anaemia

LAST

L **L**oss in weight
A **A**ngular stomatitis (cheilitis)
S **S**kin lemon-tinted (mild jaundice)
T **T**ongue is red and sore (glossitis)

Vitamin B$_{12}$ deficiency

PECS

P **P**eripheral neuropathy
E **E**yes: optic atrophy
C Spinal **C**ord degeneration
S **S**enile dementia

Normocytic anaemia

Causes

ABCDE

A **A**naemia of chronic disease
B **B**one marrow failure
C **C**idney (renal) failure
D **D**estruction of RBCs (haemolysis)
E **E**xpecting, ie pregnancy/**E**ndocrine (hypothyroidism)

Sickle-cell disease

Definition

A chronic condition with **S**ickling of RBCs caused by inheritance of haemoglobin **S** (Hb S).

Signs

SICKLE

S **S**plenomegaly/**S**ludging
I **I**nfection
C **C**holelithiasis
K **K**idney – haematuria
L **L**iver congestion/**L**eg ulcers
E **E**ye changes

The differential white cell count

White blood cell relative concentrations:

Never **L**et **M**edics **E**ducate **B**usinessmen

N	**N**eutrophils:	65%
L	**L**ymphocytes:	25%
M	**M**onocytes:	6%
E	**E**osinophils:	3%
B	**B**asophils:	1%

Leukaemia

Symptoms and signs

LEUKEMIA

L	**L**ight skin (pallor)
E	**E**nergy decreased/**E**nlarged spleen, liver, lymph nodes
U	**U**nderweight
K	**K**idney failure
E	**E**xcess heat (fever)
M	**M**ottled skin (haemorrhage)
I	**I**nfections
A	**A**naemia

Spleen

Dimensions, weight, surface anatomy

1, 3, 5, 7, 9, 11

1, 3, 5	Spleen dimensions are **1** inch × **3** inches × **5** inches
7	Weight is **7** ounces
9, 11	It underlies ribs **9** through **11**

Function

3Ps

P **P**hagocytosis of old RBCs and platelets
P **P**rotective – immunological function as it filters encapsulated organisms eg pneumococcus
P '**P**ool' of blood from which cells can be rapidly mobilised

Splenomegaly

Causes

CHINA

C **C**ongestion – portal hypertension
H **H**aematological – haemolytic anaemia, sickle cell disease
I **I**nfection (eg malaria, EBV, CMV, HIV)
N **N**eoplasia – CML, myelofibrosis, lymphoma
A **A**utoimmune – RA, sarcoidosis, amyloidosis

Massive splenomegaly causes

Massive – **M**yelofibrosis
          CML
          Malaria

Splenectomy indications

TIAs

T **T**rauma
I **I**TP
A **A**naemic – haemolytic
S hyper-**S**plenism

Hodgkin's lymphoma

Classification

A   **A**symptomatic – enlarged painless nodes e.g. in neck or axillae
B symptoms   **B**ad – fevers, night sweats, weight loss, pruritis, lethargy

Staging

The Ann Arbor staging of I–IV is further subdivided into sections depending on whether:

A **A**symptomatic
B Presence of **B** symptoms
E Localised **E**xtra-nodal extension
S **S**pleen involved

Treatment

For stages III and IV, cyclical chemotherapy in the form of the **ABVD** regimen can be administered with or without adjuvant radiotherapy:

A **A**driamycin
B **B**leomycin
V **V**inblastine
D **D**acarbazine

Non-Hodgkin's lymphoma

Classification

Classified according to the **R**evised **E**uropean and **A**merican **L**ymphoma (**REAL**) classification based on clinical, biological and histological criteria.

Treatment

For diffuse large B-cell lymphoma, the **CHOP** regimen may be used:

C **C**yclophosphamide
H **H**ydroxy daunorubicin
O **O**ncovincristine
P **P**rednisolone

Thrombocytopenia

Causes

PLATELETS

P Platelet disorders: TTP, ITP, DIC
L Leukaemia
A Anaemia
T Trauma
E Enlarged spleen
L Liver disease
E Ethanol
T Toxins: benzene, heparin, aspirin, chemotherapy.
S Sepsis

Immune thrombocytopenic purpura (ITP)

Causes

MAID

M Malignancy
A Autoimmune diseases: SLE, thyroid disease, RA
I Infections: malaria, EBV, HIV/Idiopathic (commonest cause)
D Drugs, eg quinine

Symptoms

BBC

B Bruising
B Bleeding: mucosal and nasal
C Cycles heavy; menorrhagia

Differentials

MAM

M Myelodysplasia
A Acute leukaemia
M Marrow infiltration

Myeloproliferative disorders

Polycythaemia

Signs and symptoms

HIGH Hb

H Headaches
I I-sight blurry/Itching
G OverGrown spleen; splenomegaly
H Hearing problems; tinnitus
H Hypertension
b breathlessness

Polycythaemia rubra vera

Signs and symptoms

PolyCythaemia Rubra Vera **(PCRV)**

P Plethora/Pruritis
C Cyanosis
R Ringing in ears
V Vision blurred

Complications

THUGS

T Thrombosis; stroke, MI
H Haemorrhage; resulting from defective platelet function
U Peptic Ulceration
G Gout
S Renal Stones

Disseminated intravascular coagulation (DIC)

Causes

CLOTS (as this is a disorder of the clotting cascade)

C **C**ancer/**C**omplications from pregnancy, eg missed miscarriage, severe pre-eclampsia, placental abruption, amniotic emboli
L **L**iver disease (severe)
O Haemangi**O**mas
T **T**rauma (surgery)
S **S**epsis (Gram-negative infection)

Complications

SALT

S **S**hock
A **A**cute renal failure/**A**RDS
L **L**ife-threatening haemorrhage
T **T**hrombosis with organ ischaemia/infarction

Multiple myeloma

Symptoms

BIG or BAK (take your pick!)

B **B**one pain: often in back and ribs
I **I**nfections: often recurrent
G **G**eneral: tiredness, thirst, polyuria, nausea, constipation, mental change (resulting from $\uparrow Ca^{2+}$)

B **B**ack pain
A **A**naemia
K **K**idney insufficiency

(Usually presents with the triad of **BAK**)

Management

First line is the **ABCM** regimen; or the **VAD** regimen can be followed:

A **A**driamycin
B **B**leomycin
C **C**yclophosphamide
M **M**elphalan

V **V**incristine
A **A**driamycin
D **D**examethasone

Complications

FRCS & P

F **F**ractures: pathological
R **R**enal failure (in up to one-third of patients)
C **C**arpal tunnel syndrome
S **S**pinal cord compression
P **P**olyneuropathies

Myelodysplasia

Five subgroups: 4 **R**s and 1 **C**

R **R**efractory anaemia
R **R**efractory anaemia with ring sideroblasts (RARS)
R **R**efractory anaemia with excess blasts (RAEB)
R **R**AEB in transformation (RAEB-t)
C **C**hronic myelomonocytic leukaemia (CMML)

Symptoms of bone marrow failure; **BEDRooM** (50% are diagnosed after routine blood count)

B **B**ruising
E **E**pistaxis
D **D**izziness
R **R**ecurrent infections
M **M**alaise

Signs of bone marrow failure

PIPES

P	**P**allor
I	**I**nfections
P	**P**urpura
E	**E**cchymoses
S	**S**ystolic flow murmur

Immunosuppressive drugs

PC PAM

P	**P**rednisolone
C	**C**iclosporin
P	Cyclo**P**hosphamide
A	**A**zathioprine
M	**M**ethotrexate

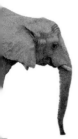

8. Infectious diseases

Diseases and conditions

Common cold (coryza)

Rhinoviruses are usually the cause, remember that a **Rhino**ceros has a large nose, and colds tend to produce a mucopurulent nasal discharge.

Gastroenteritis

Causes

LESS GERMS

L   *Listeria*
E   *Escherichia coli*
S   *Staphylococcus aureus*
S   *Salmonella*
G   *Giardia lamblia*
E   *Entamoeba histolytica*
R   **R**otavirus
M   **M**ushrooms
S   *Shigella*

Hepatitis

Viral hepatitis transmission routes

Hepatitis **A** and **E** transmitted by the f**AE**cal–oral route

Hepatitis **B** and **C** transmitted by **B**lood products and **C**exual intercourse amongst other routes

HIV

Groups at high risk of developing infection

HIV

H	**H**omosexuals/**H**aemophiliacs
IV	**IV** drug abusers

Infectious mononucleosis

Glandular fever

Typically affects young adults and is also known as the kissing fever because it is spread by saliva or droplets. It is caused by the Epstein–**Barr** virus: if your parents find out you have this you might get **BARR**ed from going out.

Leprosy

Clinical presentation

LEProsy

L	**L**oss of sensation in affected skin/**L**oss of function (paralysis)
E	**E**nlargement of affected superficial nerves (tender too)
P	**P**ositive identification of *M. leprae* under microscope

Malaria

Four plasmodium types produce disease

F.VOM

F	*Falciparum*
V	*Vivax*
O	*Ovale*
M	*Malariae*

Common early symptoms

Heard **A M**osquito

H	**H**eadache
A	**A**norexia
M	**M**yalgia/**M**alaise

Common later symptoms

Feel Rather Cold

F **F**ever (peaks every third day, ie tertian)
R **R**igors
C **C**hills

Signs

HAJ

H **H**epato-splenomegaly
A **A**naemia
J **J**aundice

Complications of P. falciparum malaria

MALARIA

M **M**etabolic (lactic) acidosis
A **A**ltered consciousness levels; Confusion → coma (cerebral malaria)
L **L**ungs; pulmonary oedema
A **A**naemia
R **R**educed glucose; hypoglycaemia
A **A**RF from ATN

Management

PQRST

P **P**aracetamol for fever
Q **Q**uinine
R **R**esistant malaria should be treated with mefloquine
S **S**ponging
T **T**ransfuse if severe anaemia

Pyrexia of unknown origin (PUO)

Causes

MID TUM

A PUO is defined as a fever lasting longer than 3 weeks (PUO has 3 letters) that defies diagnosis after a week in hospital

M **M**ultisystem diseases, eg connective tissue diseases; RA, SLE, PAN
I **I**nfections eg TB, endocarditis, osteomyelitis
D **D**rug fever
T **T**umours, especially lymphomas
U **U**nknown
M **M**iscellaneous diseases eg alcoholic hepatitis, factitious fever

Tetanus

Tetanus (sounds like Tightness!)

Causes **tightness** of muscles, muscle spasm and rigidity, including locking of the jaw. The causative factor is *Clostridium tetani*'s exotoxin.

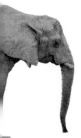

9. Neurology

Anatomy

Cranial bones

These are annoying so can be remembered as the **PEST OF 6**

P **P**arietal
E **E**thmoidal
S **S**phenoid
T **T**emporal

O **O**ccipital
F **F**rontal

6 This indicates the number of bones

Cranial nerves

Old favourites that have been modified slightly to be less offensive!

Ooh, **O**oh, **O**oh **T**o **T**ouch **A**nd **F**eel **V**ery **G**ood **V**elvet. **S**uch **H**eaven!

O **O**lfactory (1)
O **O**ptic (2)
O **O**culomotor (3)
T **T**rochlear (4)
T **T**rigeminal (5)
A **A**bducens (6)
F **F**acial (7)
V **V**estibulo-cochlear (8)
G **G**lossopharyngeal (9)
V **V**agus (10)
S **S**pinal accessory (11)
H **H**ypoglossal (12)

Some **S**ay **M**oney **M**atters **B**ut **M**y **B**rother **S**ays **B**ig **B**rains **M**atter **M**ost

The above is arranged for the cranial nerves 1–12 in determining whether they are **S**ensory, **M**otor or **B**oth.

Branches of the facial nerve

To **Z**anzibar **B**y **M**otor**c**ar

T **T**emporal nerve
Z **Z**ygomatic nerve
B **B**uccal nerve
M **M**arginal mandibular nerve
C **C**ervical nerve

Peripheral nervous system

Neurological conditions require good understanding of the anatomy of the central and peripheral nervous systems, hence remember the order of examining the peripheral nervous system as an abnormality in each area may indicate a specific anatomical problem:

I Try to **P**ractise **R**egularly to **S**ecure **C**ool **G**rades

I **I**nspect
T **T**one
P **P**ower
R **R**eflexes – starting at the ankle, work your way up to triceps. Nerve roots are as follows:

S**1/2** – ankle
L**3/4** – knee
C**5/6** – supinator (brachioradialis) and biceps
C**7/8** – triceps

S **S**ensation
C **C**o-ordination / **C**lonus
G **G**ait

Clinical conditions

Stroke

Risk factors

MR SHAHED (the co-author of this book)

M **M**ale gender
R **R**ace
S **S**moking
H **H**ypertension
A **A**ge/**A**trial fibrillation / ↑↑ **A**lcohol
H **H**yperlipidaemia
E **E**xercise ↓ and unhealthy **E**ating
D **D**iabetes mellitus/**D**rugs (anticoagulants, cocaine)

Investigations

The 4 Ps

P **P**lasma: FBC, U&E, ESR, glucose, lipids
P **P**ump, ie heart (ECG, echocardiogram)
P **P**ipes: carotid Doppler ultrasound
P **P**icture of brain: CT/MRI; detects ischaemia or haemorrhages

Differentials to consider

MICE

M **M**S
I **I**ntracranial tumour
C **C**hronic subdural haematoma
E **E**ncephalitis

Management

ABCDEFGHI

A **A**dvice – lifestyle changes eg stop smoking, reduce alcohol intake, lose weight
B **B**P control
C **C**holesterol control
D **D**M control
E **E**lastic stockings (prophylaxis for DVT, PE)
F **F**ibrillation (anticoagulate, rate control and cardiovert as required)
G **G**uardian drugs (aspirin, ACE inhibitors, etc)
H **H**elp from occupational therapy (OT), speech and language therapy (SALT) and specialist stroke nurse
I **I**ncontinence care and limit **I**mmobility (pressure sores and contractures may develop otherwise)

Headache differentials

Acute

TICOS

T **T**rauma to head
I **I**nfection: meningitis/encephalitis
C **C**erebrovascular event: subarachnoid haemorrhage, intracranial haemorrhage/infarction
O **O**cular: acute glaucoma
S **S**inusitis

Chronic or recurrent

> **CT/MR**I (useful investigations in determining cause of headache)
>
> **C** **C**luster headaches
> **T** **T**ension headache/**T**emporal arteritis
> **M** **M**igraine/**M**edications – GTN, nifedipine, substance withdrawal
> **R** **R**aised intracranial pressure: tumour, hydrocephalus, cerebral abscess

Meningitis

Aetiology

Bacterial

> **NHS**
>
> **N** *N*eisseria meningitides (children and adults; meningococcus)
> **H** *H*aemophilus influenzae (children)
> **S** *S*treptococcus pneumoniae (adults and elderly)
> (**S**treptococcus produces the **S**everest meningitis)

Viral

> **V MECH**
>
> **V** **V**ZV
> **M** **M**umps
> **E** **E**nterovirus/**E**BV
> **C** **C**oxsackie virus types A and B
> **H** *H*aemophilus influenzae/**H**IV/**H**SV

Fungal

> **2 Cs**
>
> **C** *C*ryptococcus (associated with HIV infection)
> **C** *C*andida

Hospital-acquired (nosocomial) and post-traumatic

SPEK

S *S*taphylococcus aureus
P *P*seudomonas aeruginosa
E *E*scherichai coli
K *K*lebsiella pneumoniae

Risk factors

CHASSIS

C **C**losed communities, eg dormitories, schools, day centres/ **C**SF shunts
H **H**ead injury; basal skull fractures
A **A**lcoholism
S **S**eptic site; distant (pneumonia) or near (sinusitis; mastoiditis; otitis media)
S **S**plenectomy
I **I**mmunodeficiency
S **S**ickle cell anaemia/**S**urgery; intracranial or spinal

Migraine

Features

EAT FUN

E **E**pisodic
A **A**ura – zigzag lines
T **T**hrobbing headache
F **F**amily history/**F**(p)hoto-phobia
U **U**nilateral
N **N**ausea and vomiting

Triggers

CHOCOLATES

CH **CH**eese/**CH**ocolate
O **O**CP
C **C**affeine (or its withdrawal)
OL Alcoh**OL**
A **A**nxiety/stress
T **T**ravel
E **E**xercise
S **S**leep disturbance

Vertigo

Differentials

VOMITUS

V **V**estibular neuronitis (acute labyrinthitis)
O **O**totoxicity; aminoglycosides
M **M**énière's disease (vertigo, tinnitus, hearing loss)/**M**otion sickness
I **I**nfarction/TIA
T **T**rauma/**T**umour
U **U**nmyelination; MS
S **S**pinning (benign positional vertigo)

Raised intracranial pressure (↑ ICP)

Causes

CHIMP

C **C**SF ↑, ie hydrocephalus
H **H**aemorrhage; extradural, subdural, subarachnoid
I **I**njury to head/**I**diopathic, ie benign intracranial hypertension
M **M**eningoencephalitis
P **P**rimary or metastatic tumours

Signs in advanced stage

PEAC (remember as: ↑ ICP is at the peak of the body)

P   **P**upils: fixed and dilated/no retinal vein **P**ulsation on fundoscopy/**P**apilloedema
E   **E**xtensor posture
A   **A**pnoea and Cheyne–Stokes breathing
C   **C**ushing's reflex:

3 Bs

BP ↑
Bradycardia
Breathing shallow

Parkinson's disease (PD)

Signs and symptoms

4 Ss

S   **S**hakes – resting 'pill rolling' tremor in hands
S   **S**tiffness – rigidity; ↑ tone (lead pipe rigidity), with superimposed tremor (cogwheel rigidity)
S   **S**lowness of movement; bradykinesis
S   **S**tooped, 'simian', small-stepped gait with reduced arm swinging (festinant gait)

History

History from a PD patient should determine whether difficulties exist in the following areas:

CRAM

C   Getting in and out of a **C**hair
R   **R**olling over in bed at night
A   **A**ctivities of daily living, eg bathing and dressing oneself (buttons and shoelaces in particular)
M   **M**icrographia; smaller hand-writing

Complications

4 Ds

D **D**epression
D **D**ementia
D Autonomic **D**ysfunction: postural hypotension, constipation, urinary retention or overflow incontinence, erectile dysfunction
D **D**eath (usually from pneumonia or PE)

Multiple sclerosis (MS)

Signs and symptoms

DEMYELINATION

D **D**iplopia/**D**ysmetria/**D**ysdiadochokinesis/**D**epression
E **E**ye movement painful; optic neuritis
M **M**otor: weakness, spasticity
Y N**Y**stagmus
E **E**levation in temperature; Uhthoff's phenomenon: classic description is 'unable to get out of a hot bath'
L **L**hermitte's phenomenon: electric-shock-like sensations down the back, and sometimes the thighs on bending the neck
I **I**ntention tremor
N **N**europathic pain – trigeminal neuralgia, dysaesthesia
A **A**taxia
T **T**alking is slurred; dysarthria
I **I**mpotence
O **O**veractive bladder – urinary urgency
N **N**umbness: pins and needles (sensory)

Epidemiology

MS

MS is a feminine title (**Ms.**) hence this condition is predominantly in females (2:1 ratio)

Epilepsy

Seizures: causes

GRAND MAL

G **G**lucose ↑ or ↓
R **R**aised BP; malignant hypertension, eclampsia
A **A**lzheimer's disease
N **N**eurological problems: trauma, tumour, infection (meningitis), encephalitis, inflammation (vasculitis, MS), cerebrovascular disease
D **D**rugs – phenothiazines, tricyclics, cocaine; alcohol or benzodiazepine withdrawal
M Other **M**etabolic reasons: calcium ↓, hypoxia, porphyria
A **A**bnormal sodium: ↑ or ↓
L **L**iver failure

Remember though often no cause is found, therefore **idiopathic**

Types

Partial seizures

- Seizure localised to discrete **Part** of cortex; symptoms depend on region involved

Generalised seizures

- **Tonic** (stiffness) clonic (jerking) (**G**rand mal): **G**in & **Tonic**
- Absence (**petit** mal): usual onset in children (4–12 years), ie **petit** persons
- **My**oclonic: involuntary jerking, described by a patient as '**my** flying-saucer epilepsy', as crockery that happened to be in the hand would take off

Oxford Handbook of Clinical Medicine, pg 378, Longmore, M., Wilkinson, I., Rajagopalan, S., 6th edition.

Diagnosis

Obtain history from a witness as well as the patient

Ask witness, during typical attack

4 Fs & 2 Ts

F **F**ainting; does patient lose consciousness?
F **F**unny movement? Floppy or stiff? ie **F**itting
F **F**aecal and urinary incontinence?
F **F**ace colour changes?

T **T**ongue biting?
T **T**ime scale of attack?

Before attack

WC

W **W**arning? eg typical epileptic aura
C **C**ircumstances in which attacks occur? eg whilst watching TV

After attack

3Ms

M **M**emory? How much does patient remember about the attack afterwards?
M **M**uscle pain after attack – suggests tonic/clonic seizure
M **M**ixed-up (confused) or sleepy; post-ictal

Peripheral neuropathy

Most common causes

MADD

M **M**alignancy
A **A**lcohol
D **D**M
D **D**rugs eg anti-epileptics, anti-psychotics

Summary of all causes

ABCDEFGH

A **A**lcohol/**A**myloid
B Vitamin $B_{1, 6, 12}$ $\downarrow$
C **C**onnective tissue disorders/**C**ancer
D **D**M/**D**rugs
E **E**verything else!
F **F**riedreich's ataxia
G **G**uillain–Barré syndrome
H **H**ereditary motor sensory neuropathy (HMSN = Charcot–Marie–Tooth disease)

Diagnosis confirmation of **NE**uropathy

N **N**erve conduction studies
E **E**lectromyography

In 40% no cause is identified, despite full investigation

Cerebellar signs

DANISH GP

D **D**ysdiadochokinesis; poor rapid alternative movements
A **A**taxia (truncal)
N **N**ystagmus
I **I**ntention tremor
S **S**canning or **S**lurred speech; ask patient to say 'British Constitution'
H **H**ypotonia
G **G**ait abnormality; exaggerated broad based
P **P**ast pointing; dysmetria

Gait abnormalities

PC SHAW

P **P**arkinsonian
C **C**erebellar ataxia
S **S**pasticity
H **H**emiparesis
A **A**taxic (sensory)
W **W**addling; proximal myopathy

Motor neurone disease (MND)

Upper motor neurone (UMN) signs

Remember that everything goes **up**: **Hyper**tonia, **Hyper**reflexia, **up-going** plantar responses; Babinski's sign

Lower motor neurone (LMN) signs

Remember that everything goes **down**: **Hypo**tonia, **flaccid** weakness (muscle strength decreases), **depressed** or absent reflexes

Neurofibromatosis (NF)

Diagnostic criteria

For NF1 (von Recklinghausen's disease)

CAFÉ SPOT

C	**C**afé-au-lait spots: ≥ 6 macules of > 5 mm (children) or > 15 mm (adults)
A	**A**xillary or inguinal region freckling
F	≥2 neuro**F**ibromas of any type or 1 plexiform
É	**E**yes: ≥2 lisch nodules on iris
S	**S**keletal deformities
P	**P**ositive family history of NF1 in first-degree relative
OT	**O**ptic **T**umour; glioma

(Diagnosis is made if two of the above are found).

Differentials to consider

MUM

M	**M**cCune–Albright syndrome
U	**U**rticaria pigmentosa
M	**M**ultiple lentigenes

Myotonic dystrophy

Associated features

ABCDE

A **A**rrhythmias/**A**pathy look – facial appearance
B **B**aldness (frontal)
C **C**ardiomyopathy/**C**holecystitis
D **D**iabetes mellitus
E **E**ndocrine: hypogonadism/**E**yes: cataracts

Symptoms

PUPS

P **P**rogressive weakness (hands, legs, sternomastoids) and myotonia
U **U**nable to release grip from hand shake (worse in cold conditions)
P **P**sychiatric: mental impairment
S **S**ymptoms of associated conditions, eg cataracts, testicular atrophy

Examination

On examination remember to look for myopathic facies

5 Ss

S **S**narl
S **S**mile is poor
S WhiStling difficult
S **S**ad look
S **S**agging (drooping) mouth

Guillain–Barré syndrome

Features

4As

A **A**cute inflammatory demyelinating polyneuropathy
A **A**scending paralysis
A **A**utonomic neuropathy
A **A**rrhythmias

Remember that all myopathies are proximal except **myotonic dystrophy**.

All peripheral neuropathies are distal except **Guillain–Barré**.

Types of dysphasia

BEWARE

BE Broca's = ability to speak is **B**roken (**E**xpressive dysphasia)

WARE **W**ernicke's = **AR**ticulation good but say words that don't make sense (**RE**ceptive aphasia)

Consciousness change

Causes

AEIOU TIPS

A **A**lcohol
E **E**ncephalopathy
I **I**nfection
O **O**pioid overdose
U **U**raemia

T **T**rauma
I **I**nsulin – too much or too little
P **P**sychosis
S **S**yncope

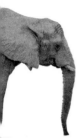

10. Obstetrics and gynaecology

Obstetrics

Anatomy

Shapes of the female pelvis

GAP

G **G**ynaecoid
A **A**ndroid/**A**nthropoid
P **P**latypelloid

This order indicates the shapes from the most common to the least common.

Pelvic dimensions

12, 13

Antero-posterior diameter: **12** cm
Transverse diameter: **13** cm

(Approximately identical for both the pelvic inlet and outlet)

Clinical conditions

Labour

Onset

Ready **M**om for **S**ome **D**iscomfort

R **R**egular and painful uterine contractions
M **M**embranes ruptured
S 'Show'
D **D**ilatation and effacement of cervix

Rate of cervical dilatation

The rate of cervical dilatation in a nulliparous woman, ie one who has never given birth to an infant capable of survival and hence this could be her **1**st pregnancy, is ~**1** cm/h.

Whereas, in a multiparous woman, ie one who has given birth to a live child after each of at least **2** pregnancies, the rate is ~ **2** cm/h.

Factors which determine the rate and outcome of labour

3Ps

P   **P**owers: strength of the uterine contractions
P   **P**assages: size of the pelvic inlet and outlet
P   **P**assengers: fetus – is it big or small, does it have anomalies, is it alive or dead?

Mechanism of delivery of the fetus

Don't **F**orget **I** **C**an **E**asily **R**uin **E**vents

Important to remember that the fetus may not always make life easy on the way out!

D   **D**escent
F   **F**lexion
I   **I**nternal rotation
C   **C**rowning of the head
E   **E**xtension of head for delivery
R   **R**estitution (external rotation of the head)
E   **E**xpulsion

Biophysical profile (BPP) constituents

Monitor **F**etuses **T**o **C**onfirm **V**iability

M   **M**ovement of fetal body
F   **F**etal breathing movements
T   **T**one of fetus
C   **C**TG monitoring for fetal heart rate
V   **V**olume of amniotic fluid

CTG interpretation

DR. C BRAVADO

DR **D**efine **R**isk – ante-partum and intra-partum history important
C **C**ontractions – is she contracting?
BR **B**aseline **R**ate – normal 110–160 beats/min
A **A**ccelerations – increase in BR by 15 beats/min or more for 15 s or longer
VA **VA**riability – 10–25 beats/min seen in normal babies
D **D**ecelerations – decrease in BR by 15 beats/min or more for 15 s or longer
O **O**verall view

Malpresentation causes

Fetuses **O**ccasionally **M**al**P**resent

F **F**etal abnormality, eg neural tube defects, hydrocephalus, neuromuscular defects
O **O**bstruction of lower uterine segment, eg due to placenta praevia, pelvic mass, fibroids, ovarian cysts
M pre-**M**aturity
P **P**olyhydramnios

Forceps and ventouse delivery: indications for use

FORCEPS

F **F**ully dilated cervix
O **O**rientate in lithotomy position
R **R**uptured membranes
C **C**ontracting uterus/**C**atheter to empty bladder
E **E**ngagement of head: at or below the ischial spines
P **P**resentation suitable: occiput
S **S**everity of pain reduced, ie pudendal, epidural, caudal analgesia

Shoulder dystocia management

HELPER

H Call for **H**elp
E **E**pisiotomy
L **L**egs up (McRoberts position)
P **P**ressure supra-pubically (not on fundus)
E **E**nter vagina for shoulder rotation
R **R**each for posterior shoulder and deliver posterior shoulder/**R**eturn head into vagina (Zavanelli manoeuvre) for C-section

Caesarean section complications

The order of all the potential complications can be easily recalled by remembering that they are all grouped according to the same ending, ie **–ate:**

- Immedi**ate**
- Intermedi**ate**
- L**ate**
- Neon**ate**

Ante-partum haemorrhage (APH) causes

APH

A **A**bruption of placenta
P **P**lacenta praevia (or vasa praevia)
H **H**aemorrhaging from the genitourinary tract

Post-partum haemorrhage (PPH) causes

4 Ts

T **T**issue (retained placenta)
T **T**one (uterine atony)
T **T**rauma (traumatic delivery, episiotomy)
T **T**hrombin (coagulation disorders, DIC)

Amniotic fluid embolism: diagnosis

Diagnosis can be made on the basis of the characteristic triad of:

3 Cs

C **C**yanosis
C **C**ollapse
C **C**lotting disorder (DIC)

Multiple pregnancy complications

This is best understood by appreciating that a multiple pregnancy usually constitutes triplets and twins, hence:

3 Ps and **2 As**

P **P**olyhydramnios
P **P**re-eclampsia
P **P**re-term labour
A **A**bortion (miscarriage)
A **A**PH

Pre-eclampsia

Classical triad witnessed

PRE

P **P**roteinuria ++
R **R**ising blood pressure – generally >140/90 mmHg
E O**E**dema

Complications

DRCOG (**D**iploma from **R**oyal **C**ollege of **O**bstetricians and **G**ynaecologists)

D **D**IC leading to HELLP
R **R**enal failure
C **C**erebral haemorrhage
O **O**ligohydramnios
G Intrauterine **G**rowth retardation (IUGR)

(HELLP**:** Haemolysis, Elevated Liver enzymes, Low Platelets)

Placenta praevia

A typical presentation of this condition is during an APH in the third trimester and is classically seen as **P**ainless **P**er **V**aginal bleeding and hence can be remembered from its title, ie **P**lacenta **P**rae**V**ia.

Complications

APH (seen again!)

A **A**PH
P **P**lacenta accreta
H **H**aemorrhaging risk increased

Polyhydramnios causes

DR. GUS

D **D**iabetes
R **R**hesus disease
G **G**I tract obstruction in fetus due to gastroschisis, exomphalos, oesophageal/duodenal atresia
U **U**rine output ↑, eg due to macrosomia
S **S**wallowing poor due to neuromuscular problems

Ectopic pregnancy risk factors

ECTOPIC

E Previous **E**ctopic/**E**ndometriosis
C **C**ontraception – IUCD, POP
T **T**ubal surgery
O **O**ther surgeries – appendicectomy, laparotomy
P **P**ID
I **I**nfertility treatment: IVF, GIFT, ZIFT
C **C**an't find a predisposing cause in 50%

Miscarriage (spontaneous abortion)

Causes and risk factors

MISCARRIAGE

M **M**ultiple pregnancy/**M**aternal disease, eg SLE, anticardiolipin antibodies, anti-phospholipid syndrome

I **I**nfections: *Salmonella*, *Listeria*, CMV, HSV, BV, etc/**I**diopathic (25% cases)

S **S**ytotoxic drugs, ie poisons

C **C**ervical incompetence (late miscarriage)

A **A**natomical anomaly, eg uterine septum

R **R**ising age of mother

R **R**adiation

I **I**mplantation of placenta abnormal (IUCD, low implantation)

A **A**bruption of placenta

G **G**enetic abnormality in fetus (aneuploidy, balanced translocation)

E **E**ndocrine: PCOS, luteal insufficiency, DM, thyroid disease

Abdominal pain: causes during pregnancy

IT ACHES

I **I**nitiation of labour

T **T**orsion – ovarian cyst (can also rupture)/uterine/**T**umour – ovarian

A **A**bruption of placenta/**A**ppendicitis/**A**bortion (miscarriage)

C **C**holestasis

H **H**aematoma of the rectus sheath

E **E**ctopic pregnancy/**E**ndometriosis

S **S**mooth muscle tumours of the uterus, ie fibroids

Gynaecology

Clinical conditions

Dysmenorrhoea

When recalling the difference between the timing of primary and secondary dysmenorrhoea, the following algorithm may be handy:

	Start	Menstruation		Resolves
		Before	After	
1° dysmenorrhoea	**1** day	<	>	2 days
2° dysmenorrhoea	**2–3** days	<	>	@ start

Dysfunctional uterine bleeding (DUB)

Three major causes

DUB

D **D**isturbed corpus luteum activity (prolonged or insufficient) – ovulatory cause (80% cases)
U **U**novulatory (10% cases)
B **B**irth control pills (as progesterone:oestrogen ↑)

Endometriosis

Symptoms

Classic 'quartet' of **DIPS**

D **D**eep dyspareunia
I **I**nfertility
P **P**elvic pain (cyclical)
S **S**econdary dysmenorrhoea

Fibroids

Symptoms

Although 50% are asymptomatic, symptoms may exist: **AM PM**

A **A**bdominal pain/swelling
M **M**enorrhagia
P **P**ressure symptoms – urinary frequency, tenesmus, oedema of leg
M 2° Dys**M**enorrhoea

Risk factors

BONE

B **B**lack women
O **O**besity
N **N**ulliparity
E **E**xpecting – ↑ growth in pregnancy

Conversely, the following ↓ risk

SMOC

S **S**moking
M **M**ultiparity
OC **O**ral **C**ontraceptive pill

Menorrhagia

Causes

BLEEDERS

B **B**leeding disorders
L **L**eiomyomas; fibroids
E **E**ndometrial polyps
E **E**ndometriosis
D **D**rugs, eg anticoagulants/**D**UB (50% cases)
E **E**ndometrial hyperplasia/carcinoma
R **R**UQ pain that can develop in PID, which may lead to menorrhagia
S **S**afe sex using an IUCD, but this device can cause menorrhagia

Menopause

Symptoms

FSH > 20 **IU/L**

Remembering that this is the most accurate blood test in confirmation of the menopause!

F   hot **F**lushes/**F**emale genitalia (vaginal) dryness and burning
S   **S**weats at night
H   **H**eadaches
I   **I**nsomnia
U   **U**rge incontinence
L   **L**ibido decreases

Long-term effects

CONU

C   **C**ardiovascular disease: IHD, stroke, arterial disease
O   **O**steoporosis: accelerated bone loss leading to osteoporosis and pathological fractures
N   **N**eurological: Alzheimer's disease
U   **U**rogenital atrophy: ↓ pelvic floor muscle tone

Hormone replacement therapy (HRT)

Pros and cons

Remembering from the above **CONU** that HRT will protect against the onset of these conditions but bearing in mind that this method of treatment does have side effects:

BEV

B   **B**reast cancer risk ↑
E   **E**ndometrial cancer risk ↑
V   **V**enous thromboembolism (DVT) risk ↑

Infertility

Causes and risk factors

INFERTILE (in females)

I **I**diopathic
N **N**o ovulation – PCOS, menopause, pituitary disease, thyroid disorders
F **F**ibroids – physical hindrance
E **E**ndometriosis
R **R**egular bleeding pattern disrupted – oligo/amenorrhoea
T **T**ubal disease leading to blocked/damaged cilia
I **I**ncreasing age >35 years
L **L**arge size – obesity
E **E**xcessive weight loss – anorexia nervosa

DO TRY CHAPS (in men)

D **D**rugs – anabolic steroids, cannabis, cocaine, sulfasalazine, colchicines, nitrofurantoin, tetracycline, alpha and beta blockers
O Epididymo-**O**rchitis/**O**bstruction of epididymis or vas deferens
T **T**rauma to testes
R **R**etrograde ejaculation
Y C**Y**stic fibrosis
C **C**hromosomal abnormalities/varico**C**ele
H **H**igh sitting testes, ie undescended
A **A**ntisperm antibodies
P **P**ost-pubertal mumps orchitis
S **S**perm abnormalities:

- Azoospermia: absent
- Oligospermia: ↓ numbers
- Teratospermia: abnormal morphology
- Asthenospermia: abnormal motility

Utero-vaginal prolapse

Predisposing factors

PROLAPSE

P   **P**regnancy (multiparity, baby >4.0 kg)
R   **R**ace (more likely in white women)
O   **O**estrogen deficiency
L   **L**abour (prolonged second stage, pushing before fully dilated, instrumental delivery)
A   **A**natomy (short vagina)
P   **P**elvic surgery
S   **S**train on supports (chronic cough, constipation, heavy lifting, obesity)
E   **E**lastin and collagen abnormalities (eg Ehlers–Danlos syndrome)

Prolapse classification

Classified according to degree and anatomical site

VIP

1st degree: descent of cervix within **V**agina
2nd degree: descent of cervix to **I**ntroitus
3rd degree: descent of cervix outside introitus; **P**rocidentia

Types

TUCRE

T   U**T**erine
U   **U**rethrocele
C   **C**ystocele
R   **R**ectocele
E   **E**nterocele

Urge incontinence (detrusor instability or overactivity)

Pathophysiology

Urge to **U**rinate followed by **U**ncontrollable complete emptying of bladder due to detrosor muscle being **U**nstable

Symptoms

Must remember that there are psychological sequelae of incontinence, hence is not a **FUNI** condition

FUNI

F Urinary **F**requency
U **U**rgency
N **N**octuria
I **I**ncontinence

Uro-dynamic stress incontinence (genuine stress incontinence)

Pathophysiology

Sphincter incompetence leads to leakage of small amounts of urine on **S**tress ie on **S**neezing, **S**tanding, laughing and coughing.

Symptoms

UFOs

U **U**rge incontinence/**U**rgency
F **F**requency
O feeling of 'some **O**bject coming down' if associated with prolapse
s **s**tress incontinence

Pelvic inflammatory disease (PID)

Too not **M**anage **PID(D) CAN** be **LETHAL**

Symptoms

T **T**emperature >37°C
M **M**enorrhagia
P **P**elvic pain (chronic)
I **I**ncreased vaginal discharge
D **D**eep dyspareunia
D **D**ysmenorrhoea (2°)

Causes

C *C*hlamydia trachomatis
A **A**ctinomycetes
N *N*eisseria gonorrhoeae

Complications

L Lose ability to conceive, ie inferility
E Ectopic pregnancy risk ↑
T Tubal blockage
H Hydrosalpinx (fallopian tube has inflammatory exudates)
A Asherman's syndrome/Abscess in pelvis
L Liver-to-bowel adhesions may develop, ie Fitz–Hugh–Curtis syndrome

Post-coital bleeding

Causes and risk factors

5 Cs

C Cervical carcinoma
C Cervical erosion
C Cervical polyps
C Cervicitis
C Recent Colposcopy
C *Chlamydia* infection

Ovarian carcinoma

Risk factors

↑ PERIODS

P Parity none or low
E Early menarche
R Race – white Caucasian
I Infertility
O Ovulation induction using drugs (over a long time period)
D Delayed menopause
S Socioeconomic status: high

Endometrial carcinoma

Risk factors

NOT LUMP ie uterus is enlarged and irregularly softened

N **N**ulliparity
O **O**besity
T **T**amoxifen therapy
L **L**ate menopause
U **U**nopposed oestrogen therapy
M Diabetes **M**ellitus
P **P**COS/**P**ersonal or family history of breast or colon cancer

Cervical intraepithelial neoplasia (CIN) and cervical carcinoma

Risk factors

Early **S**ex can **S**eriously **H**arm **H**er

E **E**arly sexual activity
S **S**moking
S **S**ocioeconomic status: low
H **H**PV infection
H **H**IV infection

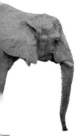

11. Ophthalmology

Anatomy and histology

Posterior = Puny

Posterior chamber is **smaller** in size than the anterior chamber:

Anterior chamber

Between cornea and iris

Posterior chamber

Between iris and lens

Aqueous humour

Aqueous humour flows from posterior to anterior chamber through the canal of Schlemm

Vitreous humour

Vitreous humour is posterior to the lens

Iris

RS

Radial **S**mooth muscle fibres (dilator pupillae), supplied by **S**ympathetic nervous system

AP

Annular smooth muscle fibres (sphincter pupillae), supplied by **P**arasympathetic nervous system, from Edinger–Westphal nucleus and CN III

The optic disc; macula

The blind spot is not hard to miss as it is marked with an X! The blind spot is in the centre of the optic disc, which is paler than the surrounding pink of the retina. The optic disc is the area of the retina that marks the head of the optic nerve. This is in the inferomedial part of the eyeball. The blind spot is the point where the central artery and vein divide into four parts in an X shape.

The fovea centralis is approximately 4 mm lateral to the optic disc and is the most photosensitive part of the retina; together with its surrounding area it constitutes the macula. Light from objects fall upon the macula and allows vision to occur.

Retinal layers

Outer layer – pigment layer, contains melanocytes and is reflective

Inner layer – **neural** layer

Deepest layer – rods and cones

- Rods – black and white
- **Co**nes – **Co**lour vision

Optic nerve, chiasma, tract

The optic nerve travels through the optic tracts. Another x-shaped structure; optic chiasma, is formed by the two optic nerves, which pass backwards from the eyeballs to meet in the midline beneath the brain.

Diseases and conditions

Allergic eye disease

HFS

H	Delayed **H**ypersensitivity
F	Hay**F**ever conjunctivitis
S	**S**pring catarrh

Hayfever conjunctivitis

ACE

A **A**llergic history (usually to animal dander or pollens)
C **C**hemosis and lacrimation of eye
E **E**ye is red and itchy

Blepharospasm

4Bs

B Often preceded by exaggerated **B**linking
B Begins unilaterally, becomes **B**ilateral
B Can lead to **B**lindness
B Symptoms managed by **B**enzhexol and **B**otulinum toxin

Blindness and partial sight

Worldwide causes of blindness

CAT

C **C**ataracts (accounts for 50% of world blindness)
A Vitamin **A** deficiency
T **T**rachoma

Risk factors for cataract

DEHYDRATION

D **D**M/**D**ehydration crises
E **E**ye diseases: glaucoma, uveitis
H **H**ypertension/**H**ypocalcaemia
Y D**Y**strophia myotonica
D **D**iet being poor in β-carotene and antioxidants
R **R**ace and family history
A **A**ccidents/**A**lcohol excess
T **T**oxicity (steroids, etc)/**T**oxoplasmosis/**T**obacco smoke
I **I**onising radiation
O **O**ld age
N **N**o protective factors (eg oestrogens, prophylactic aspirin use)

Ophthalmoscopic classification of cataracts

3Rs

R ImmatuRe cataracts
RR Red Reflex still occurs

Dense cataracts – no red reflex

Clinical presentation of conjunctivitis

BURN

B Burning and lacrimation along with itching and possibly photophobia
U Usually bilateral, if unilateral consider another differential diagnosis
R Red and inflamed conjunctiva, eyelids may be stuck together with purulent discharge
N Normally self-limiting, can be treated with antibiotics

Diabetes mellitus and the eye

The diabetic eye

Spots, Dots and Blots

Spots Cotton wool spots (ischaemic nerve fibres)

Dots and **Blots** Background retinopathy = **D**ots (microaneurysms) + **B**lots (haemorrhages due to rupture of microaneurysms)

Diabetic maculopathy

Macula becomes damaged and oedematous due to leakage from vessels close to it.

Proliferative retinopathy (PR)

Retina and optic disc develop thread-like blood vessels that bleed easily and damage eyesight. Maculopathy and PR can seriously damage vision.

Diplopia

Causes of uniocular diplopia

ABCD

A **A**stigmatism
B **B**ehavioural – psychogenic
C **C**ataract
D **D**islocated lens

The external eye

Entropion

(**IN**)tropion: the eyelids turn in, usually the lower lid. The eyelashes irritate the cornea.

Ectropion

(**EX**)tropion: the eyelids are **EX**posed, usually lower lid **E**version, causing eye irritation.

Glaucoma

Acute (closed angle) glaucoma

CLOSED

C **C**ornea appears hazy due to oedema
L **L**ights appear to have haloes and vision is blurred during an acute uniocular attack
O **O**ccurs due to blocked drainage of aqueous humour from the anterior chamber via the canal of Schlemm
S **S**hallow anterior chamber is a risk factor and may be noticed in the other eye
E **E**yeball feels hard due to raised intraocular pressure
D **D**ilatation of pupils at night worsens the condition

Chronic simple (open angle) glaucoma

OPEN

O **O**ptic disc pales as damage progresses (atrophy)
P **P**ressure in the eyes >21 mmHg causes optic disc cupping and capillary closure which causes nerve damage
E **E**merging from the optic disc, blood vessels appear to have breaks
N **N**asal and superior fields are lost first, with the last to go being the temporal fields

Optic atrophy

Causes

MICRO

M **M**S (demyelination)
I **I**njury
C **C**ompression, eg pituitary tumour or meningioma
R **R**aised glucose, ie diabetes/**R**aised ICP (persistent)
O Toxic, eg methan**O**l

Optic neuropathy

Signs

PLAC

P **P**ale disc
L **L**oss of visual acuity/**L**oss of red colour vision
A **A**fferent pupillary defect
C **C**entral scotoma

Papilloedema

Causes

ROHM (sounds like Rome!)

R **R**aised ICP/**R**etinal vein thrombosis
O **O**ptic neuritis
H **H**ypercapnia
M **M**alignant hypertension

Ptosis

Causes

MAM X POT

M **M**uscular dystrophy
A **A**bsent nerve to the levator muscle (congenital)
M **M**yasthenia gravis
X **X**anthelasma
P **P**oorly developed levator
O **O**edema of the upper lids
T **T**umour of the upper lids

Horner's syndrome is often the first cause to come to mind but it only causes slight ptosis

Pupils

Horner's syndrome

MATES

M **M**iosis
A **A**nhidrosis
T p**T**osis
E **E**nophthalmos
S **S**ympathetic nervous supply to iris disrupted

Causes of Horner's syndrome

PuPil SMALL

P **P**ancoast's tumour
P **P**aralysis (Klumpke's)
S **S**yringomelia in the pons
M **M**ultiple sclerosis
A **A**ortic aneurysm
L **L**esions of hypothalamus
L **L**ymphadenopathy of cervical nodes

Argyll **R**obertson pupil

The so-called prostitute's pupil, *accommodates but does not react*. Occurs in neurosyphilis and DM. There is bilateral miosis with pupil irregularity.

The red eye

Some dangerous causes of red eye

CIG (**sig**nificant)

C   **C**orneal ulcers
I   **I**ritis (acute)
G   **G**laucoma (acute)

Some easily treated causes of red eye

SEC (can be treated in a **Sec**ond – not quite!)

S   **S**pontaneous conjunctival haemorrhage
E   **E**piscleritis
C   **C**onjunctivitis

Some common causes of red eye

GO SUCK

G   **G**laucoma
O   **O**rbital disease
S   **S**cleritis
U   **U**veitis
C   **C**onjunctivitis
K   **K**eratitis

Refraction (long- and short-sightedness)

Myopia (short-sightedness)

The eyeball is too **long** – correct with con**cave** spectacle lens: 'the eyeball is **long** and has to be kept in a **cave**'

Hypermetropia (long-sightedness)

The eyeball is too **short** – correct with con**vex** spectacle lens: 'the eyeball is **short** and is **vex**ed by this'

Retinal detachment

Causes

SITS

S **S**econdary to some intraocular problem (melanoma)
I **I**diopathic
T **T**rauma
S **S**urgery for cataract

The 4 Fs of retinal detachment

F **F**loaters (small dark spots on a bright background are generally harmless)
F **F**lashes (migraine)
F **F**ield loss (dark cloud covers a field of vision)
F **F**alling acuity (serious)

Retinitis pigmentosa features

RP

R **R**etinal degeneration can occur and leads to blindness
P **P**articles of black **P**igment fleck mid and peripheral fundus

Retinoblastoma features

WHITES

W **W**hite reflex instead of the normal red reflex seen in photographs
H **H**ereditary in ~45% of cases, due to a faulty gene on chromosome 13
I **I**nflamed eye may develop
T **T**umour develops before the age of five
E **E**yes, unilateral in ~60% of cases
S **S**quint is common

Sudden painless loss of vision

FAST

F Amaurosis **F**ugax
A **A**rteriosclerotic ischaemic optic neuropathy
S **S**ubacute loss of vision – optic neuritis/**S**toppage of blood
flow in central retinal artery and retinal vein
T **T**emporal arteritis/giant cell arteritis

Squint

Non-paralytic squint (strabismus)

Exotropia, **(EX)**otropia, one eye looks **EX**ternally: divergent squint

Esotropia, **(IN)**otropia, one eye looks **IN**ternally. **Co**nvergent
squint is **Co**mmonest type in children

Management of non-paralytic squint

3 Os

O **O**ptical, spectacles are provided to correct refractive errors if
they exist
O **O**rthoptic, patch the good eye to give more practice to the
squint eye
O **O**peration, resection of the rectus muscles

Paralytic squint

Diplopia occurs when looking in the direction of the paralysed
muscle, individuals may complain of headache when repeatedly
asked to look in that direction

III nerve palsy (oculomotor)

The vagrant's palsy: eye looks down and out!

Ptosis, **P**roptosis and **P**upil is fixed and dilated

IV nerve palsy (trochlear)

Eye cannot look down and in because superior oblique is
paralysed

VI nerve palsy (abducens)

Eye is medially deviated and cannot look laterally from the midline; lateral rectus is paralysed

CN innervation of the extra-ocular muscles:

$LR_6 (SO_4)_3$

Lateral Rectus: CN6
Superior oblique: CN4
All the others: CN3

This aids in working out what direction the eye looks in dependant upon which CN palsy

Tears

Causes of excess lacrimation

FACE

F **F**oreign body or corneal abrasions
A **A**cute glaucoma
C **C**onjunctivitis
E **E**motion (typical man, I list this last!)

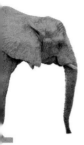

12. Paediatrics

The newborn baby

Gestation

Stillbirth	Preterm	Full-term	Post-term
Baby >24 weeks gestation, with no signs of life after delivery	<37 completed weeks	37–42 completed weeks	>42 completed weeks

Birth weight

Small for gestational age	Very low birth weight	Extremely low birth weight
Birth weight <10th centile	<1500 g	<1000 g

A trick to remember the approximate weight a child should be by their age:

[Age (in years) + 4] × 2 = weight (kg); therefore, a child of 1 should be approximately 10 kg and a child of 10 should be approximately 28 kg. (This does not work beyond 10 years of age.)

APGAR score

APGAR

The Apgar score is a scoring system devised by Dr Virginia Apgar in 1952 to identify newborns in need of immediate medical care; coincidentally her name lends itself to remembering the system. It is usually recorded at 1, 5 and 10 min after birth and is given a score of 0, 1 or 2 for each of the 5 elements.

Scores at 1 min:

7–10 ('I am normal' = 9 letters)

4–6 (ill bab = 6 letters)

1–3 (die = 3 letters), a score of 0–3 requires rapid resuscitation or they will die

Score		0	1	2
A	**A**ppearance: cyanosis – peripheral, central, none	Pallor	Body blue	Pink all over
P	**P**ulse: heart rate	Absent	<100/min	>100/min or higher
G	**G**rimace: response to stimulation	None	Grimace only	Cry
A	**A**ctivity: movement of the baby (muscle tone)	Limp	Some tone in limbs	Active movements
R	**R**espiratory rate	None	Slow, irregular	Regular, with cry

Resuscitation

Indications

IF KEMPT

I	**I**nstrumental delivery
F	**F**etal distress
K	**K**nown congenital abnormality
E	**E**mergency caesarean section
M	**M**ultiple births
P	**P**rematurity
T	**T**hick meconium stains the liquor

Evidence of severe fetal asphyxia

CARE (they require extra **care**)

C	**C**ord blood pH <7.05
A	**A**pgar score of <5 at 10 min
R	**R**espiration does not develop spontaneously beyond 10 min
E	**E**ncephalopathy develops, including abnormal neurological signs including convulsions

Death or severe handicap occurs in approximately 25% of the most severely asphyxiated term infants.

Intrauterine growth retardation (IUGR)

Symmetrical or Asymmetrical

Symmetrical growth retardation – at **S**tart or during early pregnancy, **S**mall head and **S**hort length

Asymmetrical growth retardation – **A**dvanced pregnancy, **A**bdominal growth reduced compared to head circumference (due to selective shunting of blood to the brain)

IUGR versus small for gestational age (SGA)

A baby with a birth weight below the 10th centile is SGA; this may be normal or due to IUGR

Causes of IUGR

IUGR

I   Inherited – chromosomal malformation and genetic disorders
U   Utero-placental insufficiency
G   General factors – maternal malnutrition, drugs, smoking
R   Rubella and other congenital/transplacental infections

Congenital infections that need to be screened for in severe IUGR

TORCH

T   Toxoplasmosis
O   Other (syphilis)
R   Rubella
C   CMV
H   Hepatitis, HIV

Later complications of IUGR

HID

H   Hypertension
I   Ischaemic heart disease
D   DM

Congenital abnormalities

The commonest **congenital** abnormality is **congenital** heart disease with an incidence of 8 per 1000 births.

Congenital heart diseases

Tetralogy of Fallot

SHOP

S   ventricular Septal defect (interventricular)
H   Hyper-trophy of right ventricle
O   Overriding aorta
P   Pulmonary stenosis

Cyanotic heart diseases

5 Ts

T **T**runcus arteriosus
T **T**ransposition of the great arteries
T **T**ricuspid atresia
T **T**etralogy of Fallot
T **T**otal anomalous pulmonary venous return

Common syndromes

Trisomy 13, Patau syndrome

('Patau syndrome' has 13 letters)

Trisomy **18**, Edward's syndrome

(**E**ighteen and **E**dward both begin with **E**)

Trisomy 21, Down's syndrome

Features

DOWNS

D **D**ysplastic ears/**D**ysplastic pelvis (seen on X-ray)
O **O**cciput is flat/**O**verly large tongue
W **W**idely spaced 1st and 2nd toes and a high-arched palate/**W**eak/ 'floppy' baby (hypotonia)
N **N**eck skin abundant
S **S**hort, broad hands with single palmar crease/**S**lanting eyes/ **S**peckled iris (Brushfield's spots)

Turner's syndrome (45 XO)

(Please refer to Chapter 5, Endocrinology)

VACTERL association

VACTERL

V	**V**ertebral anomalies
A	**A**nal atresia
C	**C**ardiac anomalies
TE	**T**racheo-o**E**sophageal fistula
R	**R**enal anomalies
L	**L**imb abnormalities (especially absent/small radii leading to curved and shortened forearms)

Pierre–Robin syndrome

PIERRES Chin

P	**P**roblems
I	**I**n
E	**E**ating and
R	**R**espiration
R	**R**elated to
E	**E**ye abnormality
S	**S**mall chin (micrognathia) with or without
C	**C**left palate

Cleft lip and palate

Pierre–Robin syndrome: expected problems

EUSTA

E	**E**ustachian tube dysfunction leading to conductive hearing loss (regular audiological assessments are warranted)
U	**U**nusual dentition
S	**S**peech problems
T	**T**rouble with establishing milk feeds
A	**A**spiration of milk

Surgical repair of lip is at **3** months (lip has **3** letters), repair of palate is at 9 months (palate has **6** letters, this is done **6** months after the lip correction).

Neural tube defects (spina bifida)

The defects can be divided into 4 categories:

MAMS

M **M**eningocele
A **A**nencephaly
M **M**yelomeningocele
S **S**pina bifida occulta

Congenital dislocation of the hips (CDH)

Examination

SLOB

S **S**kin creases – are they symmetrical?
L **L**eg length equal?
O **O**rtolani's test – the **O**bviously dislocated hip will not AB-Duct fully
B **B**arlow's test – the disclocata**B**le hip will give a clunking feel as it slips out of the acetabulum

Risk factors

CDH

C **C**ommoner in females
D Breech **D**elivery
H Family **H**istory

Guthrie test

Heel **P**ri**C**k (performed 5–7 days after birth to look for following conditions)

H **H**ypothyroidism
P **P**henylketonuria
C **C**ystic fibrosis

Developmental assessment

Good Father Soothes Son

Check each of these four areas:

G **G**ross motor development
F **F**ine motor development
S **S**peech and language development
S **S**ocial development

Also check hearing and vision, correcting for prematurity until the child is 2 years old. Be concerned with delay in all areas rather than delay in one area, which might be familial.

Primitive reflexes

MPRAG

M **M**oro
P **P**lacing reflex
R **R**ooting
A **A**tonic neck reflex
G **G**rasp reflex

Important milestones

Time	Gross motor development	Fine motor development and vision	Speech and language development and hearing	Social development
6 weeks		'Follow' (**6** letters) Follows objects with jerky eye movements		'Smiles' responsively (**6** letters in smiles)
6–**9** months	Props up (sits with self-propping)	'Transfers' (**9** letters) between hands	Babbling	'Strangers' (**9** letters): stranger anxiety
10–12 months	'Walks alone' (**10** letters)	'Pincer grip' (**10** letters)	'Mama, dada, no' (**10** letters)	Plays 'pattercake' (**10** letters)
18 months	Climbs stairs	Tower of 3 or 4 cubes Scribbles using fist	Points to parts of body on request	Spoon feeds, drinks from cup
2 years			Links 2 words (**2** words at **2** years) into sentences Understands **2** step commands	Learning to use potty for number 1's and number 2's (this is variable but many start at 2.5 years)
3 years	Rides a **tri**cycle		**3**-word sentences, talks a lot	Can repeat **3** digits
4 years		Draws **square**	Counts **4** objects	

Developmental warning signs

MRS

M **M**aternal concern
R **R**egression in previously acquired skills
S **S**miling not occurring by 10 weeks

Infant nutrition

Breastfeeding

Advantages

PACES (as it can be done at the mother's own pace)

P   **P**sychological satisfaction
A   **A**nti-infective property/**A**topic disorders risk ↓
C   **C**onvenient
E   **E**xpenseless, ie free
S   **S**timulates growth and development

Disadvantages

KIDS

K   vitamin **K** deficiency in breast-milk
I   **I**nfection transmission risk eg HIV
D   **D**rugs excreted in milk
S   **S**tressful and tiring for mother

Contraindicated drugs in breast-feeding

BREAST

B   **B**romocriptine
R   **R**adiation
E   **E**thosuxamide/**E**rgotamine
A   **A**miodarone
S   **S**ex hormones/**S**timulant laxatives
T   **T**etracycline

Formula milk feeds

Preparation

SAMS Formula Feed

S **S**terilise feeding bottle
A **A**dd appropriate volume of cooled boiled water to the bottle
M **M**ilk powder is added to the water (1 level scoop to each 30 ml of water)
S **S**hake bottle well
F **F**ridge until ready to feed
F **F**eeding time, rewarm the feed to room temperature or body temp before feeding (not in microwave)

Weaning

4–**6** months	Pureed foods ('pureed' has **6** letters)
6–**9** months	'Finger eat' (**9** letters) (finger foods)
9–12 months	Eat 'three meals' (**10** letters so at – **10** months)
>12 months	Undiluted full-fat pasteurised cow's milk in beaker, adult food chopped-up

Acute presentations – the acutely ill child

Four main modes of presentation of serious illness in children

SURE

S **S**hock
U **U**nconscious/drowsy/fitting child
R **R**espiratory distress
E **E**mergencies (surgical)

Shock

Causes

BASHED

B	**B**urns (fluid loss)/**B**lood loss
A	**A**naphylaxis
S	**S**eptic shock (meningococcal septicaemia), toxic shock syndrome
H	**H**eart failure
E	**E**lectric shock
D	**D**KA

Clinical features

TRUMP

T	**T**achycardia /**T**achypnoea
R	**R**estlessness/capillary **R**efill is prolonged
U	**U**rine output reduced
M	**M**etabolic acidosis
P	**P**ulse is thready/**P**ale skin

Unconscious/drowsy/fitting child

Rapid assessment of level of consciousness

AVPU

A	**A**lert?
V	Responds to **V**oice?
P	Responds to **P**ain?
U	**U**nresponsive?

Meningitis

Please refer to Neurology, Chapter 9

Brain tumours

Clinical presentation

BAN HENS

B **B**lurred vision
A **A**taxia (clumsiness)
N **N**ystagmus
H **H**eadache
E **E**ndocrine dysfunction
N **N**ausea and vomiting
S **S**quint (6th nerve palsy)

Febrile fits

4 Fs

F **F**ever >39°C
F **F**itting
F **F**ainting, loss of consciousness
F **F**lushing and sweating – pallor, cyanosis or flushed

Acute lymphoblastic leukaemia (ALL)

ALL

A **A**naemia/thrombocytopaenia/**A**ching in bone
L **L**ymphadenopathy
L **L**ethargy/malaise

Respiratory failure

Causes

PC FED BRAHMS

P   **P**neumonia
C   **C**ystic fibrosis/**C**roup
F   **F**oreign body
E   **E**piglottitis
D   **D**rug ingestion
B   **B**ronchiolitis
R   **R**aised ICP
A   **A**sthma
H   **H**ead injury
M   **M**eningitis/muscle weakness
S   **S**evere cardiac failure

Clinical features

GRINTS

G   **G**runting
R   **R**estlessness or confusion
I   **I**ntercostal recession
N   **N**asal flaring
T   **T**achypnoea
S   **S**hortness of breath

Treatment

HIT

H   **H**igh-flow oxygen
I   **I**ntubate and ventilate if rising PCO_2
T   **T**reat underlying cause

Respiratory distress

Asthma

Presentation

CWS

C   **C**ough (dry/nocturnal/worse with exercise)
W   **W**heeze
S   **S**hortness of breath

Uncontrolled asthma

SCAG

S **S**chool time off for hospital attendance (PICU)
C **C**hronic chest deformity
A **A**cute exacerbations are frequent
G **G**rowth is poor

Also see 'Chronic presentations' below for more about asthma

Pneumonia

Causes: viral

PAIR C

P **P**arainfluenza virus
A **A**denovirus
I **I**nfluenza virus
R **R**espiratory syncytial virus
C **C**oxsackie virus

Causes: bacterial

SIM

S *Streptococcus pneumoniae*
I *Haemophilus Influenzae*
M *Mycoplasma pneumoniae*

Predisposing factors

I CRICK

I **I**nhaled foreign body
C **C**ongenital anomaly of bronchi
R **R**ecurrent aspiration
I **I**mmunosuppression
C **C**ongenital cardiac problems
K **K**artagener's syndrome

Bronchiolitis

Causes

PIA

P **P**arainfluenza virus
I **I**nfluenza virus
A **A**denovirus

Points to ask in the history

WARD C

W **W**heeze
A **A**pnoea – episodes of not breathing?
R **R**espiratory distress – laboured breathing?
D **D**ifficulty feeding
C **C**ough/**C**oryza

Findings on examination and investigation

CHEW

C **C**hest X-ray may show **C**onsolidation, patchy **C**ollapse
H **H**yperinflation
E over **E**xpansion of chest
W **W**idespread **W**heezes and crackles

Pharyngitis

Causes

EARS (always check the ears in a child with a sore throat)

E **E**nterovirus
A **A**denovirus
R **R**hinovirus
S Group A β-haemolytic ***S**treptococcus*

Stridor

Causes

A CLEFT

A **A**naphylaxis
C **C**roup
L **L**aryngomalacia
E **E**piglottitis
F **F**oreign body
T **T**onsillar abscess (quinsy)

Croup

Causes

RIP

R **R**SV virus
I **I**nfluenza virus
P **P**arainfluenza virus

Epiglottitis

Clinical presentation

DOC SHOT (there are serious consequences of missing this potentially life-threatening diagnosis!)

D **D**rooling, unable to swallow
O **O**nset is sudden
C **C**ough is minimal
S **S**eptic looking child
H **H**IB vaccination is absent
O **O**lder children
T **T**alking minimal if at all

Also:

6 Ss

S **S**eptic
S **S**ilent
S **S**udden
S **S**aliva drools
S **S**wallowing difficult
S **S**wollen epiglottis

Emergencies

Intussusception

Clinical presentation

3Ss

S **S**creaming and pallor
S **S**tool has redcurrant jelly appearance
S **S**ausage-shaped mass palpable in right side of abdomen

Acute diarrhoea and dehydration

Causes of acute diarrhoea, viral

RAN

R **R**ota virus
A **A**strovirus
N **N**orwalk virus

Causes of acute diarrhoea, bacterial

CESS

C *C*ampylobacter
E *E*scherichia coli
S *S*higella
S *S*almonella

Chronic presentations

Asthma

Presentation

CWS

C **C**ough (dry/nocturnal/worse with exercise)
W **W**heeze
S **S**hortness of breath

Uncontrolled asthma

SCAG

S **S**chool time off for hospital attendance (PICU)
C **C**hronic chest deformity
A **A**cute exacerbations are frequent
G **G**rowth is poor

BTS guidelines for assessing severity of acute asthma attack

Severe attack

Can't **R**eally **T**alk **P**roperly

C **C**annot talk or feed properly due to breathlessness
R **R**espiratory rate   → >30 breaths/min in 2–5 years
                          ↳ >50 breaths/min in <2 years
T **T**achycardia   → >120 beats/min in 2–5 years
                          ↳ >130 beats/min in <2 years
P **P**EFR < 50% predicted in > 5 years

Life threatening attack

CHEST

C **C**yanosis/**C**onfusion/**C**oma
H **H**ypotension
E **E**xhaustion
S **S**ilent chest
T **T**hreatening PEFR <33% predicted in those above 5 years old

BTS guidelines for stepwise management of acute asthma attack

OBS AM

O **O**xygen – high flow via reservoir bag
B **B**ronchodilators – salbutamol nebulised or IV, ipratroium bromide via volumatic spacer
S **S**teroids – oral prednisolone or IV hydrocortisone
A **A**minophylline infusion
M **M**agnesium sulphate – *not* indicated in children at present (controversial evidence)

BTS guidelines of stepwise management of chronic asthma: children aged 5–12 years

5 Steps, hence **5Ss**

Step 1 – **S**albutamol (short-acting β_2-agonist inhaler)
Step 2 – add low dose inhaled **S**teroid eg fluticasone
Step 3 – add-on therapy: **S**almeterol (slow-acting β_2-agonist inhaler)
Step 4 – further increased dose of inhaled **S**teroids
Step 5 – add oral **S**teroids eg prednisolone

Education after acute asthma attack

NEAR

N **N**ormal activities should be maintained as far as possible
E **E**mergency protocol should be understood
A **A**dherence to medication should be stressed
R **R**ecognition of acute attacks

Diabetes mellitus

Please also refer to Endocrinology, Chapter 5

Presentation

Pee-**P**ee **W**ee

P **P**olyuria
P **P**olydipsia
W **W**eight loss over weeks

Poor diabetic control

LEG PEP

L **L**ipodystrophy, if do not rotate injection sites, leads to erratic absorption of insulin
E **E**pisodes of hypoglycaemia
G **G**rowth is poor
P **P**olyuria
E **E**pisodes of hyperglycaemia
P **P**olydipsia

Chronic diarrhoea

5Cs

Inflammatory causes of chronic diarrhoea include:

C **C**rohn's disease
C Ulcerative **C**olitis

Malabsorptive causes of chronic diarrhoea include:

C **C**ystic fibrosis
C **C**oeliac disease
C **C**ow's milk intolerance

Crohn's disease

CROHNS

C **C**hildhood presentation (late)
R **R**emissions and **R**elapses
O **O**ral/perianal ulcers and arthritis
H **H**istory of abdominal pain, anorexia, growth failure, fatigue, fever, diarrhoea
N **N**utritional programmes induce remission, elemental diets effective in severe cases
S **S**teroids/**S**ulfasalazine/**S**urgical resection for localised disease may be needed

Ulcerative colitis

ULCERS

U **U**C presents with diarrhoea with mucus and blood
L **L**iver disturbance, pain, weight loss and arthritis may occur
C **C**orticosteroid enemas or suppositories may help
E **E**xacerbations and remissions
R **R**isk of colonic cancer developing later in life
S **S**ulfasalazine is given orally and **S**urgery (colectomy) may be required in severe cases

Cystic fibrosis

Features

CF

C   **C**hest infections are common
F   **F**ailure to thrive/**F**atty stools

and:

MRS SEW

M   **M**econium ileus in 10% as neonates
R   **R**ecurrent pneumonia
S   **S**teatorrhoea/**S**(c)irrhosis of liver develops eventually
S   **S**hort stature
E   **E**xtra energy is required (40% more)
W   **W**eight gain is poor

Cerebral palsy

Associated problems

LUSH VERBS

L   **L**earning difficulties
U   **U**ndernutrition and poor growth
S   **S**peech disorders
H   **H**earing loss
V   **V**isual impairments
E   **E**pilepsy
R   **R**espiratory problems
B   **B**ehavioural disorders
S   **S**quint

Diagnosis in first year

PAM

P   **P**rimitive reflexes persist
A   **A**bnormal tone – initially decreased but then increased
M   **M**otor development is delayed

Diagnosis on clinical grounds

HAD

H **H**emiplegia
A **A**thetoid cerebral palsy
D **D**iplegia

Epilepsy

Please refer to Neurology, Chapter 9

Bedwetting

Management

PEES

P **P**ressin (desmopressin – ADH analogue)
E **E**xplanation not blame and punishment
E **E**nuresis alarm
S **S**tar chart with star for dry nights

Failure to thrive

Mild

Failure **2** thrive

Crosses **2** centile lines

Severe

Crosses 3 centile lines

Pyrexia of unknown origin (PUO)

Causes

PAIN TOUCH

Fever of one week or more duration in young children or 2–3 weeks in adolescents. They should be hospitalised and observed with blood cultures taken at fever peaks when the yield is greatest.

P **P**neumonia
A **A**bscesses
I **I**nfective endocarditis, **I**BD
N **N**eoplastic disease
T **T**B
O **O**steomyelitis
U **U**TI
C **C**ollagen vascular disease
H **H**epatitis/**H**IV

Short stature

Differential

ABCDEFG

A **A**lone (neglected infant)
B **B**one dysplasias (rickets, scoliosis, mucopolysaccharidosis)
C **C**hromosomal (Turner's, Down's)
D **D**elayed growth
E **E**ndocrine (low growth hormone, Cushing's syndrome, hypothyroid)
F **F**amilial
G **G**I disease (coeliac disease, Crohn's)

Still's disease

Features

STILLS

S **S**piking illness/**S**evere malaise
T **T**here could be myalgia/arthralgia
I **I**ncreased size of liver/spleen
L **L**ose weight, anaemia
L **L**ooks like malignancy
S **S**almon-pink rash

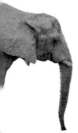

13. Psychiatry

Symptoms and signs in psychiatric disorders

Psychiatric disorders have been classified in varying ways, with different diagnoses being manipulated into hierarchies. The most widely used systematic classification of psychiatric illness is the *International Classification of Disease*, currently on its 10th revision (ICD-10). It categorises 458 mental disorders grouped into 10 major groups.

Organic, including symptomatic, mental disorders

Can be divided into **generalised** (involve entire cortex) and **focal** (involve a specific part of the cortex). Generalised can further be classified as acute brain syndrome (delirium), subacute brain syndrome and chronic brain syndrome (dementia).

Causes of delirium

DELIRIUM

D **D**egenerative
E **E**pilepsy (post-ictal states)
L **L**iver failure
I **I**ntracranial (injury to the head, subarachnoid haemorrhage, TIA, meningitis, cerebral abscess)
R **R**heumatic chorea
I **I**nfections – pneumonia, septicaemia
U **U**raemia
M **M**etabolic – electrolyte imbalance

Diagnostic criteria of delirium

C, DIPPS (dipping of consciousness)

A and 2 or more from B

A **C** **C**louding of consciousness with acute onset

B **D** **D**isorientation or impaired memory
  I **I**ncoherent speech
  P **P**erceptual disturbances such as illusions or hallucinations
  P **P**sychomotor changes, either retardation or restless overactivity
  S **S**leep is affected, with insomnia and daytime sleeping

Clinical presentation of subacute brain syndrome (delerium tremens)

C, TREMENS

C **C**louding of consciousness and disorientation
T **T**remor and agitation occur in the first 12 h of alcohol withdrawal
R **R**estlessness, insomnia and fear have a sudden and dramatic onset
E **E**pileptic seizure may occur 12–48 h after withdrawal
M **M**ovements include ataxia and tremor
E **E**xcessive sweating with tachycardia, flushing or pallor
N **N**ightmares, panic and startled reactions. May have vivid, threatening hallucinations and illusions
S **S**tricken by fear, seen especially in the facial expression

Clinical presentation of chronic brain syndrome (dementia)

Features

5As

Aphasia – mixed receptive and expressive language problems; **A-phrase-ia**

Apraxia – cannot carry out a motor task, **a-prax-ia; A-practical-ia**

Agnosia – cannot recognise people or objects, **I-knows-u?**

Causes

DEMENTIAS

D **D**iabetes/neuro**D**egenerative diseases
E **E**thanol/**E**motional (depression, anxiety, etc)/**E**lderly
M **M**edication toxicity (opiates, anti-convulsants, levodopa, sedatives)/**M**etabolic imbalance
E **E**nvironmental (eg CO poisoning)
N **N**utritional (vitamin and iron deficiencies)/**N**ormal pressure hydrocephalus
T **T**rauma/**T**umours/**T**hyroid disorders, ie hypothyroidism
I **I**nfection (meningitis, encephalitis, pneumonia, syphilis)
A **A**lzheimer's disease
S **S**troke

Focal brain syndromes

Wernicke's encephalopathy

Features

A SOAP

A **A**ltered consciousness (confusion)
S **S**ubacute brain syndrome
O **O**phthalmoplegia
A **A**taxia of gait/**A**lcoholics commonly affected
P **P**rodromal nausea may be present

Korsakoff's syndrome

Features

6 Cs

C **C**ognitive impairment revealed when acute state clears
C **C**ognitive functioning preserved
C **C**louding of consciousness does not occur
C **C**an not lay down new memories, but long-term memory is preserved
C **C**ommonly found in alcoholics due to thiamine deficiency
C **C**onfabulation (make up answers)

Causes of thiamine deficiency

CAT

C   **C**arcinoma of stomach
A   **A**naemia (pernicious)/**A**lcoholism
T   **T**oxaemia of pregnancy

Temporal lobe lesions

Temper may develop, along with personality change and unpredictable behaviour

Frontal lobe lesions

3Fs

F   **F**atuous jocularity (inappropriate mild euphoria)
F   **F**amiliarity bordering on the obscene with sexual disinhibition
F   **F**oresight is impaired

Parietal lobe lesions

Places (difficulty with orientation)

Disorders due to psychoactive substances

Alcoholism

CAGE questionnaire

C   Have you ever felt you should **Cut** down on your drinking?
A   Have people **Annoyed** you by commenting on your drinking?
G   Have you ever felt **Guilty** about your drinking?
E   Have you ever needed a drink first thing in the morning to get rid of a hangover or for nerves (**Eye opener**)?

>1 'yes' answer makes alcoholism likely

Schizophrenia and delusional disorders

Psychotic symptoms of schizophrenia can be divided into **positive** and **negative** symptoms:

Positive symptoms (sometimes called type I schizophrenic symptoms)

THREAD (they lose the **thread** of reality)

T	**T**hinking may become disturbed, neologism usage
H	**H**allucinations may occur, usually auditory
R	**R**educed contact with reality, the natural barrier between subjective and objective deteriorates
E	**E**motional control may be disturbed with inappropriate laughter or anger (incongruous affect)
A	**A**rousal may lead to worsening of symptoms
D	**D**elusions may occur

Negative symptoms (sometimes called type II schizophrenic symptoms)

LESS (patient appears **less** active)

L	**L**oss of volition, underactivity and social withdrawal
E	**E**motional flatness, lose normal modulation of mood
S	**S**peech is reduced, monosyllabic if at all
S	**S**lowness in thought and movement, psychomotor retardation may occur

Paranoid schizophrenia

PA

The commonest form of schizophrenia

P	**P**ersecutory delusions
A	**A**uditory hallucinations and other disorders of perception such as bodily sensations, and hallucinations of taste, smell and vision

Diagnostic criteria for schizophrenia

DEAD (in the absence of cerebral damage, intoxication, epilepsy or mania), one or more of the following symptoms for longer than 1 month indicates schizophrenia:

D **D**isorders of thought possession (insertion, withdrawal, broadcasting)

E **E**xperiences of passivity (other people are controlling their feelings or impulses – passivity phenomenon)

A **A**uditory hallucinations (thought echo, running commentary, being constantly referred to in the third person)

D **D**elusions that persist (culturally inappropriate)

Mood (affective) disorders

ADE

A **A**nxiety
D **D**epression
E **E**lation

Anxiety

PAD (they are anxious and **PAD** around their room)

The patient complains of:

P **P**anic attacks
A All-pervasive **A**pprehension
D Feelings of impending **D**oom

Symptoms of worry

POOR WOLF

W Symptoms of **W**orry

For worry to be abnormal: **POOR**

> **P** **P**ainful (mentally)
> **O** **O**ut of proportion
> **O** **O**ut of control
> **R** **R**ecognisable

O **O**bsessional symptoms; performing an action against conscious resistance, such as ritual hand washing; resistance brings greater mental anguish; these activities can take up hours and interfere with other daily activities
L **L**ow-mood symptoms, ie depression, with loss of ability to enjoy things
F **F**earful symptoms; fear and anxiety feel the same; a panic attack is 'sudden onset of feeling frightened or terrified for no reason.' Can happen even in a safe environment

Depression

Symptoms of depression

SLUMP

S **S**uicidal ideation or plans
L **L**ack of interest, enjoyment (anhedonia), energy, appetite or libido
U **U**nworthiness
M Early **M**orning waking
P **P**oor concentration/**P**sychomotor retardation or agitation

Bipolar affective disorder (manic-depressive psychosis)

Diagnosis of a manic episode

A period of euphoria/irritability lasting for a week or more which is disruptive to social and work commitments, with at least three from the following list:

INSPIRE (often go through a creative splurge)

I	**I**ncreased activity or restlessness
N	**N**eed for sleep is reduced
S	**S**ubjective increased speed of thought
P	**P**ressure of words
I	**I**ncreased self-esteem (grandiose ideas)
R	**R**educed inhibitions
E	**E**asily distracted

Obsessive-compulsive disorder (OCD)

The individual often feels a compulsion to carry out rituals which can take over their lives. Resisting the compulsion can lead to anxiety, although insight is not lost.

Obsessional phenomena seen in OCD

TIRED

T	**T**houghts of an unpleasant or obscene nature
I	**I**mages that are vivid and distressing/**I**mpulses that can be embarrassing
R	**R**ituals such as frequent washing/**R**uminations about minutiae
E	**E**laborate ways of carrying out tasks
D	**D**oubts and constant re-checking of items such as locks, doors, gas and electricity supplies

Personality disorders

The ICD-10 classifies personality disorders as 'Deeply ingrained maladaptive patterns of behaviour'.

Some personality disorders

SHOP DED (personalities are often deep-grained, it is hard to **shop** for a new one)

S **S**chizoid personality (emotional coldness with preference for fantasy)

H **H**istrionic personality (dramatises events, often a romantic)

O **O**bsessional personality (overly conscientious due to insecurities)

P **P**aranoid personality (excessively sensitive to perceived humiliation)

D **D**ependent personality (lacks personal resources, seeks constant reassurance)

E **E**motionally unstable personality disorder (explosive temper with minimal provocation)

D **D**issocial personality (psychopathic personality – lacks empathy for others, impetuousness, violence, easily frustrated)

Suicide

Risk factors

SAD PERSONS

S **S**ex (male)

A **A**ge (older)

D **D**epression

P **P**revious attempt

E **E**xcessive alcohol or substance abuse

R **R**ational thinking, loss of

S **S**ickness (chronic illness)

O **O**rganised plan

N **N**o social supports

S **S**tated intention to self-harm

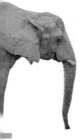

14. Renal

Renal histology and anatomy

- The human kidneys are bean-shaped and measure 10–12 cm in length, 5–6 cm in width and 3–4 cm in depth
- The outer parenchymal **C**overing is called the **C**ortex and the **M**iddle is called the **M**edulla
- They are retroperitoneal and are situated on either side of the vertebral column, at the level of T12–L3
- The transpyloric plane (**L1**) goes through the hilum of only **1** kidney, and it's the **L**eft one; this is because the right kidney is about 1.5 cm lower than the left
- Both move 3 cm up and down with respiration.

The functional unit of the kidney is the nephron, which consists of:

- a glomerulus
- a proximal tubule
- a loop of Henle
- a distal tubule
- a collecting tube

Each kidney contains approximately 100,000 nephrons.

The renal arteries

The common way of remembering the branches of the renal arteries is by crossing your hands at the wrist so that the palms face you. The thumbs and fingers represent the following segments:

Thumb   The single posterior segment branch
Forefinger   The apical segment
Middle finger The upper segment
Ring finger   The middle segment
Little finger The lower segment

Ureter to ovarian/testicular artery relation

Water under the bridge

The **ureters** (which carry water), are **posterior** to the ovarian/testicular artery. This is clinically important, since a common surgical error is to cut the ureter instead of the ovarian artery when removing the uterus.

Role of the kidneys

REEM (it does **reams** and **reams** of work)

R **R**egulates: fluid balance/acid–base balance/electrolyte balance
E **E**ndocrine: erythropoietin/prostaglandins
E **E**xocrine: waste products/drugs
M **M**etabolic: vitamin D/PTH

Diseases and conditions

Acute renal failure (ARF)

Detection of ARF

ACUte

A **A**cute presentation over hours or days
C **C**reatinine rises
U **U**rea rises (±oliguria <400 ml/24 h)

Causes of ARF

ACUte

A **A**TN/**A**cute GN
C **C**irculatory dysfunction ie shock – hypovolaemia, sepsis, cardiogenic
U **U**rinary outflow obstruction

Causes of ARF on anatomical lines

Pre-renal failure (PRF)	*Renal disorder*	*Urinary obstruction*
Kidney is structurally normal but functionally abnormal	**Structural abnormalities in the kidney**	**ARF develops only if there is bilateral obstruction**
Renal hypoperfusion (shock – hypovolaemia, sepsis, cardiogenic), renal artery stenosis, the hepatorenal syndrome	Acute tubular necrosis (ATN) following shock, acute glomerulonephritis, HUS, exogenous nephrotoxins, endogenous nephrotoxins	Stone, ureteric obstruction by pelvic malignancy, bladder outflow obstruction, retroperitoneal disease (retroperitoneal fibrosis, lymphoma)

Management of ARF

AEIOU and manage complications

A **A**ssess intravascular volume status, if volume depleted (pulse increased, BP decreased, postural hypotension, low JVP, cool peripheries), or overloaded (pulse has gallop rhythm, BP increased, raised JVP, basal crepitations, peripheral oedema), correct as appropriate

E **E**mpirical treatment with antibiotics if patient is septic, remove IV and catheter when not required to prevent sepsis. Also **E**ject nephrotoxic medications from patient's drug regimen

I **I**n and out, place a central line and urinary catheter, match input to losses with 500 ml for insensible losses with additional 500 ml if pyrexial. Daily fluid balance chart and weight chart

O **O**ral nutritional intake should be monitored, high calories are needed (>2000 kcal/day) and high proteins (0.5–1 kg/day) but less if dialysis is unavailable. Possibly nasogastric tube

U **U**rinary obstruction should be identified and removed

Complications of ARF

HOB

H **H**yperkalaemia/**H**TN
O Pulmonary **O**edema
B **B**leeding

Acute tubular necrosis (ATN)

ATN is usually associated with circulatory problems, and **RAN**:

R **R**habdomyolysis
A **A**bnormalities of urinary system suggestive of tubular dysfunction
N **N**ephrotoxins (**TA³N** – **T**etracyclines, **A**minoglycosides, **A**CE inhibitors, **A**mphotericin B, **N**SAIDs)

Chronic renal failure (CRF)

Definition

Irreversible, substantial, long-standing loss of renal function

Common causes

ACID and BASE

A **A**nalgesic nephropathy
C **C**ystic disease (PCKD)/Chronic GN and Pyelonephritis
I **I**nterstitial nephritis
D **D**M/**D**rugs: ACE inhibitors, NSAIDs, Gentamicin

B **B**P ↑
A renal **A**rtery atheromatous disease
S **S**tones (nephrolithiasis)
E **E**nlarged prostate

Uncommon causes

SMASH

S **S**LE
M **M**yeloma
A **A**myloidosis
S **S**cleroderma
H **H**US

Severity of CRF

Glomerular filtration rate (ml/min)	Severity of renal failure
30–50	Mild
10–29	Moderate
<10	Severe
<5	End-stage renal failure (results in death without renal replacement therapy)

Clinical presentation of CRF

RESIN & 8 Ps

R **R**etinopathy
E **E**xcoriations (scratch marks)
S **S**kin is yellow
I **I**ncreased blood pressure
N **N**ails are brown
P **P**allor
P **P**urpura and bruises
P **P**ericarditis and cardiomegaly
P **P**leural effusions
P **P**ulmonary oedema
P **P**eripheral oedema
P **P**roximal myopathy
P **P**eripheral neuropathy

Late clinical presentation of CRF

CASE

C **C**oma
A **A**rrhythmias
S **S**eizures
E **E**ncephalopathy

Management of CRF

AB_2CD_2E

A **A**naemia – exclude other causes (iron deficiency, chronic infection) and then treat with EPO
B **B**P control – ACE inhibitors (caution with renal artery stenosis)/**B**one disease of renal cause (osteodystrophy) – Treat as soon as ↑ PTH. ↓ dietary phosphate (less milk, cheese, eggs) and use phosphate binders eg Calcichew®
C **C**alcium – maintain serum levels with vitamin D analogues eg alfacalcidol and calcium supplements as this ↓ risk of bone disease and risk of ↑ PTH (2° & 3°)
D **D**iet – 'Renal' diet: high energy intake, however restriction of protein, potassium, phosphate and salt. Foods that are restricted/ excluded include: chocolate, coffee, banana, fruit drinks and dairy products
D **D**rugs – avoid nephrotoxic drugs and NSAIDs
E o**E**dema – diuretics eg furosemide and metolazone

Differentiating between nephrotic and nephritic syndrome

Ne**PHrO**tic syndrome (**P**roteinuria and **H**ypoalbuminaemia and **O**edema)

Ne**PH**ritic syndrome (**P**roteinuria and **H**aematuria)

Nephr**O**tic syndrome has the **O** and the marked **O**edema

Do not get the 2 Hs in the syndromes mixed-up, remember that the oedema is due in part to the hypoalbuminaemia but may also be seen in nephritic syndrome. However, the H in nephritic syndrome indicates haematuria.

Nephrotic syndrome

HOP

H **H**ypoalbuminaemia (<30 g/l)
O **O**edema
P **P**roteinuria (>3 g/24 h)

Causes of nephrotic syndrome

GASH'D

G **G**N
A **A**myloidosis
S **S**LE
H **H**enoch–Schonlein purpura (HSP)
D **D**M/**D**rugs – gold, penicillamine, captopril, NSAIDs

Clinical features of nephrotic syndrome

HE, FAX

H **H**ypertension
E **E**ffusions (pleural)
F **F**acial swelling/'**F**rothy' urine
A **A**scites
X **X**anthelasma/**X**anthomata

Clinical findings of nephrotic syndrome

Protein LEAC

L **L**ipids up
E o**E**dema
A **A**lbumin down
C **C**holesterol up

In nephrotic syndrome, the **proteins leak** out

Complications of nephrotic syndrome

SALT

S **S**usceptible to infections (peritonitis)
A **A**RF
L **L**oss of low-molecular-weight binding proteins in urine/ hyper-**L**ipidaemia
T **T**hromboembolism (DVT, PE, renal vein thrombosis)

Management of nephrotic syndrome

BAD HIP

B **B**ed rest, monitor U&E, BP, fluid balance, weight
A **A**nticoagulation with heparin (5000 U/12 h)
D **D**iuretics (furosemide ± metolazone or spironolactone)/**D**iet: avoid excess protein
H **H**ypertension and **H**yper-lipidaemia should be treated
I **I**nfections should be treated before they gain dominance
P **P**roteinuria should be treated in those with CRF with ACE inhibitors or spironolactone

Nephritic syndrome

Common causes of nephritic syndrome

PAIRS

P **P**ost-streptococcal GN
A **A**lport's syndrome
I **I**gA nephropathy
R **R**PGN
S **S**LE

Oliguria

Urine output <400 ml/day and is normally due to drinking less water or being hot.

Abnormal causes of oliguria

3Rs

R   **R**enal perfusion is decreased
R   **R**enal parenchymal disease
R   **R**enal tract obstruction

Polyuria

Polyuria is excretion of larger than normal volumes of water and is normally due to drinking large amounts of water.

Pathological causes of polyuria

3Ds

D   **D**iabetes mellitus
D   **D**iabetes insipidus
D   **D**isorders of renal medulla (failure to concentrate urine)

Renal pain

Causes

R. PAIN

Dull constant pain felt in loin

R   **R**enal obstruction (there may be swelling and tenderness)
P   **P**olycystic kidney disease (PCKD)
A   **A**cute pyelonephritis
I   Renal **I**nfarction
N   Acute **N**ephritic syndrome

Clinical presentation of ureteric pain (renal colic)

WARS

W   **W**axes and wanes
A   **A**ssociated with fever and vomiting (often)
R   **R**adiates to abdomen, groin or upper thigh
S   **S**evere loin pain

Causes of ureteric pain (renal colic)

RCS, Renal **C**olic **S**evere

R **R**enal stones
C **C**lot
S **S**loughed papillae

Urine dipstick: common items detected on urinalysis

Have **G**ood **L**ong **P**ee **K**idneys **N**ice

H **H**aematuria (blood)
G **G**lucose
L **L**eucocytes
P **P**roteinuria
K **K**etones
N **N**itrites

Haematuria

Renal causes of haematuria

PIST

P **P**olycystic kidney disease/**P**apillary necrosis
I **I**gA nephropathy/**I**nterstitial nephritis/**I**nfections (TB, cystitis, pyelonephritis, Bilharzia)
S **S**tones
T **T**rauma/**T**umour

Extrarenal causes of haematuria

MIST

M **M**alignancy (bladder, prostate, urethra)
I **I**nfection (cystitis, prostatitis, urethritis)
S **S**ickle-cell disease/**S**tones
T **T**rauma

Haematuria – all causes grouped together

HAEMATURIA

H   **H**ereditary (polycystic kidney disease)/**H**SP
A   Ig**A** nephropathy
E   **E**mbolism (infective endocarditis)
M   **M**alignant HTN
A   **A**cute and chronic glomerulonephritis
T   **T**umours/**T**rauma/**T**oxic drugs
U   **U**rolithiasis
R   **R**enal papillary necrosis
I   **I**nfection (pyelonephritis, cystitis, prostatitis, urethritis)
A   **A**nticoagulants

Proteinuria

Renal causes of proteinuria

HUGOS

H   **H**US
U   **U**TI
G   **G**N
O   **O**rthostatic proteinuria
S   **S**LE

Extrarenal causes of proteinuria

DEEP

D   **D**M
E   **E**xercise
E   **E**jaculation (recent)
P   **P**regnancy

Causes of glucose in the urine

DRIPS

D   **D**M
R   **R**enal tubular damage/C**R**F
I   **I**nfection
P   **P**regnancy
S   **S**epsis

Urinary tract infections

Bacteriuria (bacteria in the urine; may be asymptomatic or symptomatic)

UTI-causing microorganisms or **UTI** (presence of a pure growth of >10^8 colony-forming units/ml).

Infections of the urinary tract

Bladder	(cystitis)
Prostate	(prostatitis)
Kidney	(pyelonephritis)

Abacterial cystitis (the urethral syndrome)

One-third of symptomatic women do not have bacteriuria.

Complicated and uncomplicated UTIs

Uncomplicated UTIs have a normal renal tract and function.

Complicated UTIs

MARIO

M **M**ale patients
A **A**bnormal renal tract
R **R**enal function is impaired
I **I**mpaired host defences
O **O**rganism that is virulent

Risk factors for UTIs

UTIs

U **U**rinary tract obstruction or malformation
T **T**he menopause
I **I**ntercourse (sexual)/**I**nstrumentation/**I**mmunosuppression
S female **S**ex/**S**tones

Recurrence and relapse of UTI

Recurre**N**ce of UTI is a further infection with a **N**ew organism (**N**)

Relap**S**e of UTI is a further infection with the **S**ame organism (**S**)

Organisms that cause UTIs

KEEPS

(*E. coli* is by far the commonest cause with >70% in the community and <41% in hospital)

K *K*lebsiella species
E *E*nterococcus faecalis
E *E*nterobacter species
P *P*seudomonas aeruginosa/*P*roteus mirabilis
S *S*taphylococcus saprophyticus/*S*erratia marascens

Clinical presentation of UTIs

F PUSH (there is an urgency to **PUSH** urine out with increased frequency)

F **F**requency
P **P**ain (suprapubic) on passing urine
U **U**rgency
S **S**trangury
H **H**aematuria

Advice to prevent UTIs

ADVICE

A **A**dvise women to wipe from front to back to prevent infections
D **D**ouble voiding (go again after 5 min)
V **V**oid urine after intercourse
I **I**ncrease fluid intake
C **C**ranberry juice (evidence is not impressive)
E **E**ncourage to urinate frequently

Causes of sterile pyuria

PUBIC

(Do not discount renal TB)

P **P**apillary necrosis from analgesic excess
U **U**TI with fastidious culture requirement
B **B**ladder tumour
I **I**nadequately treated UTI/**I**nterstitial nephritis
C **C**hemical cystitis, eg from cytotoxics/**C**alculi (prostatitis)/**C**ystic disease (PCKD)

Acute pyelonephritis

FLAVOR (kidneys are the only part of the urinary tract that people like to eat)

F **F**ever
L **L**oin pain and tenderness
A **A**RF
V **V**omiting
O **O**liguria (if ARF)
R **R**igors

Glomerulonephritis (GN)

GN

G **G**lomerular bleeding is indicated by haematuria with red cell casts in the urine
N **N**ephrotic syndrome/**N**ephritic syndrome presentations may occur or the individual could be asymptomatic

Subgroups of GN

- IgA Nephropathy
- HSP
- Minimal change GN
- Focal segmental glomerulosclerosis
- Mesangial nephropathy
- Proliferative GN

Clinical presentation of IgA nephropathy (Berger's disease)

NEPHRO

N **N**ephrotic syndrome
E **E**specially young males
P **P**haryngitis is associated
H **H**ypertension/**H**aematuria (recurrent macroscopic)
R **R**enal failure – occasionally/**R**apid **R**ecovery
O **O**therwise known as Berger's disease

Henoch–Schönlein purpura (HSP)

HSP

H **H**as a propensity to develop after a throat infection and affects young boys
S **S**ystemic version of IgA nephropathy (Berger's disease)
P **P**urpura (**P**urple spots do not disappear on **P**ressure) found especially over buttocks

Hydronephrosis

Differentials of unilateral hydronephrosis

PACT

P **P**elvic–uretric obstruction (congenital or acquired)
A **A**berrant renal vessels
C **C**alculi
T **T**umours of renal pelvis

Differentials of bilateral hydronephrosis

SUPER

S **S**tenosis of the urethra
U **U**rethral valve
P **P**rostatic enlargement
E **E**xtensive bladder tumour
R **R**etro-peritoneal fibrosis

Polyarteritis nodosa (PAN)

Clinical presentation

PAN

P **P**ericarditis/**P**roteinuria and renal failure
A **A**neurysms/**A**bdominal pain/**A**rthralgia along with general malaise and weight loss
N **N**ecrotising vasculitis causes aneurysms of medium-sized arteries

Adult polycystic kidney disease

Adult polycystic kidney disease (APKD), renal signs

CHURCH

C **C**ysts with renal enlargement
H **H**aematuria/**H**TN
U **U**rinary tract infection
R **R**enal failure
C Renal **C**alculi
H **H**as need of dialysis?

APKD, extra-renal signs

CALM

C **C**olonic diverticulosis
A **A**neurysms (intra-cranial) → Sub-arachnoid haemorrhages
L **L**iver cysts
M **M**itral valve prolapse

The genetic basis of APKD

ADult polycystic kidney disease is **A**utosomal **D**ominant

'Polycystic kidney' has **16** letters and is due to a defect on chromosome **16**

Dialysis

Indications for dialysis

AEIOU

A **A**cid–base problems (severe acidosis or alkalosis)
E **E**lectrolyte problems (hyperkalaemia)
I **I**ntoxications
O **O**verload, fluid
U **U**raemic symptoms

Or

SHARPE

S **S**everity of condition increases
H **H**yperkalaemia persistent (K$^+$ >7 mmol/l)
A **A**cidosis is metabolic and worsening (pH <7.2 or base excess <−10)
R **R**efractory pulmonary oedema
P **P**ericarditis (uraemic)
E **E**ncephalopathy (uraemic)

Haemodialysis (HD)

HAD

H **H**ospital or **H**ome-based
A **A**rteriovenous fistula is created at the wrist
D **D**iffusion of solute across semi-permeable membrane

Problems with HD

HD

H **H**ypotension
D **D**isequilibrium syndrome

Haemofiltration (HF)

H **H**ospital or **h**ome-based, **H**aemofilter is used and blood is filtered across this highly permeable synthetic membrane via ultrafiltration rather than diffusion
F **F**luid replacement is of an equal volume to the ultrafiltrate and there is no exposure to dialysis fluid

Problems with HF

HF

H **H**igher cost than haemodialysis
F **F**iltration is time consuming

Continuous ambulatory peritoneal dialysis (CAPD)

CAPD

C **C**APD uses smallest volume of dialysate fluid to prevent uraemia
A **A**llows patient to carry out treatment at home
P **P**eritoneum acts as semi-permeable membrane
D **D**ialysate is replaced with fresh fluid once chemical equilibrium is reached

Automated peritoneal dialysis (APD)

APD

A **A**utomated, makes use of cycler machine
P **P**atient-friendly and easy to perform
D **D**iabetes patients, those with cardiovascular disease and the elderly are advised to use this technique rather than haemodialysis

Problems with peritoneal dialysis

PD

P **P**eritonitis
D **D**ecreased efficiency (in comparison to haemodialysis)

Complications of dialysis

CHAIR (a lot of dialysis time is spent sedentary)

C **C**ardiovascular disease
H **H**ypertension
A **A**naemia
I **I**nfections
R **R**enal bone disease

Renal transplants

Contraindications for renal transplants

CASH

C **C**ancer
A **A**ctive infection
S **S**evere heart disease
H **H**IV

Complications following renal transplants

ART

A **A**theromatous vascular disease (leading cause of death)
R **R**aised BP
T **T**hrombosis (vascular)/**T**-cell immunity is immunosuppressed and leads to infections

Prostatitis

STUB (because the prostate feels like a little stub on PR)

S **S**ymptoms are flu-like
T **T**ender prostate
U **U**rinary symptoms are few
B **B**ackache of lower back

Urinary tract malignancies

Renal cell carcinoma (RCC)

Features

RCC

R **R**enal tubule (proximal) epithelium is involved
C Renal **C**ancers are 90% RCC
C **C**linical features include haematuria, loin pain, abdominal mass, anorexia, malaise and weight loss

Transitional cell carcinoma (TCC)

Risk factors

TCC

T **T**obacco smoke
C **C**yclophosphamide and other drugs eg phenacetin
C Industrial **C**arcinogens eg azo-dyes, β-naphthalene

Prostatic cancer

Features

PROSTATE

P **P**oor stream
R **R**ectal examination reveals hard and irregular prostate
O **O**bstruction of urine
S **S**econd most common malignancy amongst men
T **T**erminal dribbling
A **A**ge-related incidence, 80% >80 years (in autopsy studies)
T **T**est is prostate specific antigen (PSA) >10 µg/l (but only 1 in 3 of those with a high PSA will have prostate cancer)
E **E**vidence-based treatment has not isolated a single curative measure, treatments include: radical prostatectomy, radiotherapy or watchful waiting with monitoring of serial PSA

Vasculitis

Features

V Blood **V**essels inflamed
A **A**utoimmune
S **S**enior citizens more commonly affected
C **C**utaneous – burst blood vessels – rash with small red
     blotches
U **U**rology – haematuria, kidney failure
L **L**ungs – haemoptysis
I **I**ll health – general
T **T**ired
I **I**nfection such as influenza could trigger autoimmune
     vasculitis
S **S**teroids used to treat

Eponymous syndromes

Fanconi syndrome

Features

PHANCONI

PH **PH**osphaturia
A   **A**cquired
N   **N**ormally results in type II renal tubule disease
C   **C**ystinosis
O   **O**steomalacia in adults and Rickett's in children
N   **N**ephrocalcinosis and renal calculi are almost never seen
I   **I**nherited/**I**diopathic

Goodpasture's syndrome and Wegener's granulomatosis are rare
vasculitis conditions that affect, amongst other organs, the lungs
and the kidneys.

Goodpasture's syndrome

Features

GOODPAST

G **G**lomerulonephritis
O **O**n chest X-ray – infiltrates often in lower zones
O **O**n kidney biopsy – crescentic nephritis
D **D**eath occurs in many in the first 6 months
P **P**lasmapheresis may help in treatment
A **A**nti-basement membrane antibody is the cause of this **A**utoimmune condition
S **S**hortness of breath and **S**putum that is bloody along with a cough are common lung symptoms
T **T**reatment is with vigorous immunosuppressive treatment

Wegener's granulomatosis

Features

WEGENERS

W **W**egener's is potentially fatal
E **E**pistaxis – nasal ulcers
G **G**eneralised necrotising arteritis and **G**lomerulonephritis are a diagnostic criterion
E **E**ar – otitis media/**E**ye signs – proptosis, ptosis, conjunctivitis
N **N**ecrotising granulomas in the respiratory tract are diagnostic criterion
E **E**qually occurring in males and females
R **R**espiratory tract primarily affected (sinus, nose, trachea and lungs) and the kidneys
S High-dose **S**teroids backed up by cyclophosphamide used in treatment

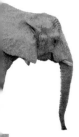

15. Respiratory

Diseases and conditions

Acute respiratory distress syndrome (ARDS)

Definition

ROAR

- **R** **R**educed lung compliance
- **O** **O**edema, non-cardiogenic pulmonary
- **A** **A**cute respiratory failure
- **R** **R**efractory hypoxaemia

Causes

ARDS

- **A** **A**spiration-gastric/**A**cute pancreatitis/**A**mniotic fluid embolus
- **R** **R**aised ICP/**R**espiratory tract infection – pneumonia
- **D** **D**KA/**D**IC/**D**rugs
- **S** **S**epsis/**S**hock/**S**moke inhalation/**S**evere burns

Asthma

Definition

CRAB

- **C** **C**hronic inflammatory airway disease
- **R** **R**eversible airway obstruction
- **A** **A**irway hyper-responsiveness
- **B** **B**ronchial inflammation

Aetiology, genetic factors

PA (as in dad)

P   **P**ositive family history
A   **A**topy

Aetiology, environmental factors

ASTHMA

A   ***A****spergillus fumigatus* spores
S   **S**moke (cigarette)
T   Respiratory **T**ract infection
H   **H**ouse dust mite
M   **M**anual work exposure to epoxy-resins, isocyanates
A   **A**nimals (furs) or pollen exposure

Aetiology, precipitating factors

ICED (remember cold)

I   **I**nfection (viral)
C   **C**old air
E   **E**motion/**E**xercise
D   **D**rugs (beta-blockers, NSAIDs)

Risk factors

FEAR UP

F   **F**amily history
E   **E**czema
A   **A**cid reflux
R   **R**hinitis (allergic)
U   **U**rticaria
P   **P**olyps (nasal)

History

WIND (feel **winded**)

W   **W**heeze
I   **I**nterferes with schooling, exercise, sleep and work
N   **N**octurnal cough, or early morning cough
D   **D**yspnoea

Examination findings

ACCEPT

A **A**ccessory muscles used
C **C**hest hyper-inflated
C **C**yanosis (very severe cases)
E **E**xpiratory phase prolonged
P **P**olyphonic wheeze
T **T**achypnoea

For management of asthma please refer to the BTS guidelines in Chapter 12, Paediatrics.

Bronchiectasis

Definition

BBC

B **B**ronchial dilatation (chronic) with frequent . . .
B **B**acterial infections due to impaired mucociliary . . .
C **C**learance (pooling of mucus)

Causes

BRONCHIAL

B **B**ronchiolitis
R **R**A
O **O**bstruction of bronchi (foreign body, tumour)
N **N**ecrotising pneumonia
C **C**ystic fibrosis/**C**(K)artagener's syndrome
H **H**IV infection
I **I**diopathic/**I**nfections (measles, pertussis)
A **A**BPA
L **L**ow immunoglobulins

COPD

COPD is a prime example of how abbreviations are commonly used in medicine, it stands for **C**hronic **O**bstructive **P**ulmonary **D**isease. It comprises chronic bronchitis and emphysema.

COPD: blue bloater versus pink puffer

Chronic **B**ronchitis has letter **B** (and not P) so **B**lue **B**loater

Em**P**hysema has letter **P** (and not B), so **P**ink **P**uffer

This is not a reliable way of differentiating between the two conditions but is used as a rule of thumb.

X-ray findings in COPD

ABCD

A   **A**ntero-posterior diameter increases (narrow mediastinum)
B   **B**ullae/'**B**ig' lungs => Hyper-inflated: >6 ribs visible anteriorly
C   **C**ardiac silhouette elongated; heart 'hangs in the wind'
D   hemi-**D**iaphragms flattened

Cryptogenic fibrosing alveolitis (CFA)

Risk factors

SWASH OF

S   **S**moking (in 75% cases)
W   **W**ood (pine in 20% cases)
A   **A**nimal dusts
S   **S**tone cutting
H   **H**airdressing
O   **O**ccupational exposure to metals (brass, lead, steel)
F   **F**arming

Signs

3Cs

C   **C**lubbing
C   **C**yanosis
C   fine **C**repitations

Management

Can be recalled from the name **CFA**

Corticosteroids
Azathioprine

Extrinsic allergic alveolitis (hypersensitivity pneumonitis)

Risk factors

BACHS

B **B**loom on bird feathers and droppings (bird fancier's lung)
A **A**lcohol brewing process, barley or malt containing *Aspergillus clavatus* (maltworker's lung)
C **C**ompost containing thermophilic *Actinomycetes* (mushroom worker's lung)
H **H**ay that is mouldy contains thermophilic *Actinomycetes* (farmer's lung)
S **S**team or humidified air that contains bacteria and amoeba (humidifier lung)

Influenza infection

Clinical manifestations

FLU

F **F**ever
L **L**ethargy
U **U**pset appetite (nausea and vomiting)

Influenza

New strains can lead to the deaths of millions. The virus is an RNA **O**rthomyxovirus and has three subtypes: A, B and C. Type A is further subtyped by **H**aemagglutinin (**H**) and **N**euraminidase (**N**).

Major changes, antigenic **S**hift: **S**hifts you into grave hence fatal

Minor changes, antigenic **D**rift: **D**rift in and out of illness hence non-fatal

Lung cancer, non-small cell

This is **no small matter**, as it is the most common cancer in the West.

Three histological types **SmAlL** (every other letter in the word small)

S **S**quamous cell carcinoma (35%)
A **A**denocarcinoma (20%)
L **L**arge cell carcinoma (20%)

Lung cancer, small cell

Also called oat cell carcinoma based on appearance.

Symptoms

ABCDEFGH

A **A**norexia and weight loss
B **B**rachial plexus involvement (Pancoast's tumour)
C **C**ough (bovine – left recurrent laryngeal nerve involvement)
D **D**yspnoea
E **E**asily fatigued muscles
F **F**ocal neurological signs from metastases
G En**G**orgement of face (SVC compression)
H **H**aemoptysis

Pancoast's tumour: relationship with Horner's syndrome

Horner's MATES live on the **COAST**

COAST A pan**Coast's** tumour is a cancer of the lung apex that compresses the cervical sympathetic plexus, causing **Horner's** syndrome, which is **MATES**

Miosis
Anhidrosis
p**T**osis
Enophthalmos
Sympathetic nervous supply to iris disrupted

Lung cancer: main sites for distant metastases

BLAB

B **B**one
L **L**iver
A **A**drenals
B **B**rain

Obstructive sleep apnoea (Pickwickian syndrome)

Aetiology

COMA MESS

C **C**raniofacial abnormalities/**C**OPD
O **O**besity
M **M**arfan's syndrome
A **A**lcohol use before sleep
M **M**acroglossia – abnormally large tongue
E **E**nlarged tonsils or adenoids in children
S **S**moking
S **S**edative use

History

SLEEP

S **S**leep is restless
L **L**iable to be irritable
E **E**xcessive daytime sleepiness (driving risk)
E **E**pisodes of nocturnal apnoea
P **P**artner reports snoring

Pleural effusion

Signs

PLEURA

P **P**ercussion note stony dull
L **L**istening for breath sounds which are diminished
E **E**xpansion decreased
U **PU**shes trachea away
R **R**esonance (vocal) decreased/pleural **R**ub
A **A**symptomatic in some cases

Pneumonia

Risk factors

INSPIRE

I	**I**mmunosuppression
N	**N**eoplasia
S	**S**moking
P	**P**re-existing lung disease
I	**I**mmobility
R	**R**espiratory tract infection/**R**eflux disease can lead to aspiration
E	**E**lderly

Causes

Gram-negative versus Gram-positive

- Gram-**N**egatives (eg coliforms) are responsible mainly for **N**osocomial pneumonia
- Gram-positives (eg *Streptococcus pneumoniae, Staphylococcus*) are thus more responsible for community-acquired pneumonia ie **s**trep and **s**taph common in **s**ociety

Prognostic criteria for pneumonia

CURB 65

C	**C**onfusion: abbreviated mental test score ≥8
U	**U**rea >7 mmol/l
R	**R**espiratory rate ≥30/min
B	**B**lood pressure <90 mmHg systolic and/or 60 mmHg diastolic
65	Age >**65** years

Pneumothorax

Causes

AIR-TIGHT

A	**A**sthma (secondary)
I	**I**njury that penetrates chest (traumatic)
R	**R**upture of sub-pleural bleb (spontaneous)

T TB
I Lung Infection – abscess/Iatrogenic
G Growth ie lung carcinoma
H Hereditary ie cystic fibrosis
T Connective Tissue disorders eg Marfan's, Ehlers–Danlos

Presentation

P-THORAX

P Pleuritic pain in the chest
T Tracheal deviation away from pneumothorax
H Hyper-resonance to percussion
O Onset sudden
R Reduced breath sounds (and dyspnoea)
A Asymptomatic if pneumothorax small/Absent fremitus
X X-ray shows collapse

Pulmonary embolism

Please refer to Surgery, Chapter 17

Tuberculosis (TB)

Features

TB is characterised by **4 Cs**

C Cough
C Caseation
C Calcification
C Cavitation

Management of pulmonary TB

RIPES

Patients often do not take their medications appropriately therefore **DOT** (**D**irectly **O**bserved **T**herapy) can be followed:

Initial phase (2 months on three to four medications)

R **R**ifampicin
I **I**soniazid
P **P**yrazinamide
E **E**thambutol (if multi-drug-resistant TB)
S **S**treptomycin (if the initial four-drug therapy fails, use streptomycin as add-on)

Continuation phase (4 months on two medications)

R **R**ifampicin
I **I**soniazid

Pulmonary TB medication side-effects

Rifam**PICIN**, turns urine orange, **PISSIN** orange

Ethambutol, optic neuritis, **EYE**thambutol

Primary TB

Primary infection is usually **P**ulmonary.

Post-primary TB, causes of reactivation

SHADO (shadow on the lung)

S **S**teroid use
H **H**IV
A **A**ge (old)/**A**lcohol
D **D**M
O **O**thers eg malignancy, malnutrition

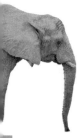

16. Rheumatology

Rheumatoid arthritis (RA)

Features

RHEUMATISM

R **R**heumatoid factor (RF) +ve in 80%/**R**adial deviation of wrist
H **H**LA-DR1 and DR-4
E **E**SR ↑/**E**xtra-articular features (restrictive lung disease, subcutaneous nodules)
U **U**lnar deviation of fingers
M **M**orning stiffness/**M**CP+PIP joint swelling
A **A**nkylosis/**A**tlanto–axial joint subluxation/**A**utoimmune/**A**NA +ve in 30%
T **T**-cells (CD4)/**T**NF
I **I**nflammatory synovial tissue (pannus)/**I**L-1
S **S**wan-neck deformity, Boutonniere deformity, Z-deformity of thumb
M **M**uscle wastage of small muscles of hand

X-ray changes

JESS

J **J**oint space loss (symmetrical)
E **E**rosion of joint
S **S**ynovial thickening
S **S**ubluxation and joint deformities

Diagnostic criteria for RA (Arthritis Research Council; ARC)

Four out of seven required.

ARMS

A **A**rthritis of >3 areas for >6 weeks in 1 year (1)/**A**rthritis of hand joints (2)

R **R**heumatoid nodules (3)/**R**adiographic changes (4)

M **M**orning stiffness for >1 h (5)

S **S**erum rheumatoid factor (6)/**S**ymmetrical arthritis (7)

Management

DMARDs (**D**isease-**M**odifying **A**nti-**R**heumatic **D**rugs)

Most **S**ufferers **C**an **G**et **A**ppropriate **P**ain **C**ontrol

M **M**ethotrexate

S **S**ulfasalazine

C **C**iclosporin

G **G**old

A **A**zathioprine

P **P**enicillamine

C Hydroxy**C**hloroquine

Felty's syndrome

Features

PANDAS

P **P**latelets ↓↓

A **A**rthritis: RA

N **N**eutropenia: ↓ WCC

D **D**ermatological problems: skin ulcers, pigmentation (particularly in lower limb)

A **A**naemia

S **S**plenomegaly

Osteoarthritis

X-ray signs

LOSS

L **L**oss of joint space
O **O**steophytes
S **S**ubchondral sclerosis
S **S**ubchondral cysts

Mono-arthritis

Differential

GO or STOP

GO GO**ut**

S **S**eptic arthritis, eg *Staphylococcus*, *Streptococcus*, Gram-negative bacilli
T **T**rauma – haemarthrosis
O **O**steoarthritis
P **P**soriatic and reactive arthritides

Poly-arthritis (eg > 2 swollen painful joints)

Differential

V**ice** P**resident'**S CARS

V **V**iruses, eg mumps, rubella, parvovirus B19, EBV, hepatitis B
P **P**ost-streptococcal reactive
S **S**pondyloarthritides
C **C**onnective tissue diseases, eg SLE
A Crystal **A**rthropathies, eg gout, CPPD
R **R**heumatoid or osteoarthritis
S **S**arcoidosis

Joint pain

Causes

ARTHRITIS

A	**A**rthritis – rheumatoid or osteoarthritis
R	**R**eactive arthritides
T	**T**endon/muscle damage
H	**H**yperuricaemia; gout
R	**R**eferred pain
I	Auto**I**mmune, eg connective tissue disease – systemic sclerosis, SLE
T	**T**umour
I	**I**schaemia
S	**S**epsis/**S**pondyloarthritides

Arthritis

Seronegative spondyloarthropathies

PEAR

P	**P**soriatic arthritis
E	**E**nteropathic arthritis (IBD)
A	**A**nkylosing spondylitis
R	**R**eiter's syndrome/**R**eactive arthritides

Ankylosing spondylitis

Features

SPINAL

S	**S**acroiliac and low back pain
P	**P**leuritic chest pain
I	**I**nherited gene marker: HLA-B27 (>90% HLA-B27 +ve, general population frequency ~ 8%)
N	**N**eck hyperextension – question mark posture
A	**A**rthritic symptoms in peripheries (asymmetrical)
L	**L**oss of spinal movement which is progressive

Extra-articular features

EXTRA

E **E**ye becomes red: anterior uveitis
X E**X**pansions of chest reduced (due to fusion of costo-vertebral joints)
T **T**horacic problem: apical lung fibrosis
R **R**egurgitation in aorta (cardiac diastolic murmur)
A **A**bdominal conditions associated with this, ie IBD

Sacroiliitis

Causes

SACRUM

S P**S**oriasis
A **A**nkylosing spondylitis
C **C**rohn's disease
R **R**eiter's syndrome
U **U**lcerative colitis
M **M**echanical causes

SLE

Diagnosis by ARA (American Rheumatism Association) criteria

(4 out of 11 of the following criteria are required to diagnose SLE)

NORA SPAHI MD

N **N**eurological abnormality – seizures/psychosis
O **O**ral ulcers
R **R**enal involvement – casts or proteinuria > 0.5g/24 h
A **A**rthritis – non-erosive
S **S**erositis – pericarditis/pleuritis
P **P**hotosensitivity
A **A**ntinuclear antibodies – +ve in 95%
H **H**aematological disorders – haemolytic anaemia or lymphopenia or thrombocytopenia
I **I**mmunological disorders – anti-dsDNA/anti-SM/anti-Ro/lupus anticoagulant/anticardiolipin
M **M**alar rash – butterfly rash
D **D**iscoid rash

Reiter's syndrome

Can't see, Can't pee, Can't climb a tree

This equates to the features of Reiter's syndrome, ie conjunctivitis, urethritis and arthritis.

CREST syndrome

Components

CREST

C **C**alcinosis
R **R**aynaud's phenomenon
E O**E**sophageal dysmotility
S **S**clerodactyly
T **T**elangiectasia

Gout

Causes and features

URATE

U **U**rate levels ↑
R **R**enal impairment hence ↓ renal excretion of urate
A **A**lcoholism
T **T**rauma precipitates gout/hyperpara**T**hyroidism
E **E**rythematous warm and tender swollen joint with ↓ range of movement and inability to bear weight. Usually MTP joint of big toe

Decreased renal excretion of urate leading to gout can be due to the following drugs:

CAN'T LEAP

C **C**iclosporin
A **A**lcohol
N **N**icotinic acid
T **T**hiazides
L **L**oop diuretics: furosemide
E **E**thambutol
A **A**spirin (low-dose)
P **P**yrazinamide

Foods that cause gout

SALTS

S **S**hellfish
A **A**nchovies
L **L**iver and kidney
T **T**urkey
S **S**ardines

Raynaud's phenomenon

Features

The mnemonic **WBC** can help you to remember the order of the skin colour changes of the fingers seen in Raynaud's:

W **W**hite – blanching of digits
B **B**lue – cyanosis and pain
C **C**rimson – reactive hyperaemia – fingers turn red in colour

Secondary causes

A Bad DOC

A **A**rterial – arteriosclerosis, thromboangiitis obliterans
B **B**lood disorders – polycythaemia
D **D**rugs – beta-blockers, OCP
O **O**ccupation – vibrating tools
C **C**onnective tissue disorders – rheumatoid arthritis, SLE, scleroderma, polyarteritis nodosa, Sjögren's syndrome

Osteoporosis

Risk factors

MR SHAHED

M **M**enopause – early
R **R**ace – white
S **S**moking/**S**lender built
H **H**istory in family
A **A**lcohol ↑↑/**A**ge ↑
H **H**igher likelihood in females
E **E**xercise – lack of/**E**ndocrine disease: Cushing's syndrome, hyperparathyroidism, acromegaly
D **D**rugs – corticosteroids, heparin, ciclosporin

Management

SCAB HER

S **S**moking cessation
C **C**alcium intake increased
A **A**ndrogens in hypogonadal men
B **B**isphosphonates

H **H**RT – oestrogen treatment
E **E**xercise
R **R**aloxifene – selective oestrogen-receptor modulator

Paget's disease

Features

BAD NEW X-RAY

B **B**one pain
A **A**pparent joint pain
D **D**eformities (bowed tibia and skull changes)

N **N**erve compression (deafness from compression of CN VIII, also affects CN II, V, VII)
E **E**levated bone blood flow (cardiac hypertrophy and high output cardiac failure)
W **W**eakness of abnormal bone leading to pathological fractures (rarely osteosarcoma develops in this condition; < 1%)

X-ray changes

- Enlargement or expansion of bone
- Osteolytic lesions
- Thickening of bone trabeculae in long bones and vertebrae
- Pseudofractures – precursor or marker for osteosarcomatous change

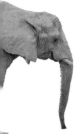

17. Surgery

Anatomy

Femoral triangle

Arrangement of contents

NAVEL – from lateral to medial, ie towards navel

N **N**erve (femoral; behind sheath)
A **A**rtery (femoral; within sheath)
V **V**ein (femoral; within sheath)
E **E**mpty space
L **L**ymphatics (with deep inguinal node)

Boundaries

Safely **I**ndicate **M**edicine **A**nd **L**imit **S**urgery

Superiorly: **I**nguinal ligament

Medially: **A**dductor longus

Laterally: **S**artorius

Retroperitoneal structures

PACKED in **R**etro-peritoneum

P **P**ancreas
A **A**orta and IVC
C **C**olon (ascending and descending)
K **K**idneys
E **OE**sophagus
D **D**uodenum (half)
R **R**ectum

Abdominal wall muscles

Spare **TIRE** around the abdomen

T   **T**ransversus abdominis
I   **I**nternal oblique
R   **R**ectus abdominis
E   **E**xternal oblique

Inguinal canal: walls

MALT: 2Ms, 2As, 2Ls, 2Ts

Start superiorly and move around in order to get posteriorly:

Roof: 2 Muscles

M   Internal oblique **M**uscle
M   Transverse abdominus **M**uscle

Anterior wall: 2 Aponeuroses

A   **A**poneurosis of external oblique
A   **A**poneurosis of internal oblique

Floor: 2 Ligaments

L   Inguinal **L**igament
L   **L**acunar **L**igament

Posterior wall: 2Ts

T   **T**ransversalis fascia
T   Conjoint **T**endon

Spermatic cord contents

The rule of 3s: 3 arteries, 3 nerves, 3 other things

3 arteries: testicular, ductus deferens, cremasteric

3 nerves: genital branch of the genitofemoral, cremasteric, autonomics

3 other things: ductus deferens, pampiniform plexus, lymphatics vessels

Layers of scrotum

Some **D**octors **E**xaggerate **C**onditions, **I**ncreasing **P**atients **V**(w)orry **T**remendously

S   **S**kin
D   **D**artos layer
E   **E**xternal spermatic fascia
C   **C**remaster muscle
I   **I**nternal spermatic fascia
P   **P**arietal tunica vaginalis
V   **V**isceral tunica vaginalis
T   **T**unica albuginea

Bowel components

Dr **J**ones **I**nvestigates **C**arefully **A**nd **C**uts **R**andomly

From proximal to distal:

D   **D**uodenum
J   **J**ejunum
I   **I**leum
C   **C**aecum
A   **A**ppendix
C   **C**olon
R   **R**ectum

Clinical conditions

Initial management of all surgical emergencies

4 As, 2 Cs, 2 Ns (could be remembered as a set of GCSE results!)

A   **A**BC assessment
A   **A**nalgesia, eg morphine
A   **A**nti-emetic
A   **A**ggressive fluid resuscitation – IV fluids and electrolyte replacement
C   **C**entral venous pressure (CVP) line – may be needed
C   **C**atheter (urinary)
N   **N**il by mouth (NBM)
N   **N**asogastric (NG) tube

Post-operative pyrexia

Causes

6 Ws

W   **W**ind: lungs are primary source of fever during the first 24–48 h; may have pneumonia
W   **W**ound: infection at surgical site
W   **W**ater: check IV line for phlebitis
W   **W**alk: DVT, due to pelvic pooling or restricted mobility related to pain and fatigue
W   **W**hiz: UTI if urinary catheterisation
W   **W**onder drugs: drug-induced fever or other allergies

Post-operative complications

General immediate

PROBS

P   **P**rimary haemorrhage/**P**ain
R   **R**eactive haemorrhage
O   **O**liguria – acute urinary retention
B   **B**asal atelectasis
S   **S**hock/**S**epsis

General early

ABCDE

A   **A**nalgesia- or **A**naesthetic-related nausea + vomiting
B   **B**reakdown of wound or anastomosis due to infection or haematoma – dehiscence / ↓ **B**P – ↓ fluid input → hypovolaemia → ↓ BP
C   **C**onfusion – acute
D   **D**VT leading possibly to PE
E   **E**levated temperature – pyrexia (*see* Causes, **6 Ws**)

General late

RIB

R   **R**ecurrence of malignancy
I   **I**ncisional hernia
B   **B**owel obstruction

Meckel's diverticulum

Rule of 2s

2 This tends to occur in **2**% of population
2 **2**:1 is the male:female ratio
2 **2** inches long
2 **2** feet from the ileo-caecal valve

Appendicitis

Differentials

When considering the diagnosis of appendicitis in women, the list of differentials can include **PMS** as these are only known to occur in women.

P **P**regnancy that could be ectopic
M **M**enstrual pains
S **S**alpingitis

Other differentials (including those occurring in both sexes)

Police **F**orce, **CID** and **M**ilitary

P **P**erforated ulcer
F **F**ood poisoning
C **C**holecystitis
I **I**BD – Crohn's disease
D **D**iverticulitis
M **M**eckel's diverticulitis

Complications

MAP

M **M**ass of appendix
A **A**bscess of appendix
P **P**erforation/**P**eritonitis

Acute pancreatitis

Causes

I GET SMASHED

I	**I**diopathic
G	**G**allstones
E	**E**thanol (alcohol)
T	**T**rauma
S	**S**teroids
M	**M**umps
A	**A**utoimmune
S	**S**corpion stings
H	**H**yperlipidaemia/**H**ypercalcaemia
E	**E**RCP
D	**D**rugs: azathioprine, diuretics

Modified Glasgow criteria for predicting severity of pancreatitis

PANCREAS

P	P_aO_2 < 8 kPa
A	**A**ge > 55 years
N	**N**eutrophils: WCC > 15×10^9/l
C	**C**alcium <2 mmol/l
R	**R**enal function: urea >16 mmol/l
E	**E**nzymes: LDH > 600 IU/L; AST >200 IU/L
A	**A**lbumin <32 g/l
S	**S**ugar: blood glucose >10 mmol/l

The presence of three or more points within the first 48 h constitutes severe acute pancreatitis and should warrant transfer to the ITU.

Management

VACCINES

V	**V**ital signs monitoring
A	**A**nalgesia/**A**ntibiotics
C	**C**atheter (urinary)/**C**alcium gluconate (if thought necessary)
C	**C**imetidine (H_2-receptor antagonist)
I	**I**V access/**I**V fluids
N	**N**BM/**N**utrition; total parenteral
E	**E**mpty gastric contents (nasogastric tube)
S	**S**urgery if required/**S**enior review

Local complications

PAIN

P **P**seudo cyst
A **A**bscesses
I **I**nfection
N **N**ecrosis

Gallstones

Risk factors

5 Fs

F **F**at
F **F**emale
F **F**orty
F **F**amily history
F **F**ertile

Complications

BECAMe **PO**r**C**elain **G**allbladder (remembering that a porcelain gallbladder is a complication of gallstones)

In the gall bladder	*In the bile ducts*	*In the gut*
BECAMe	**PO**r**C**elain	**G**allbladder
B **B**iliary colic	P **P**ancreatitis	**G**allstone ileus
E **E**mpyema	O **O**bstructive jaundice	
C **C**arcinoma		
A **A**cute and **C**hronic cholecystitis	C **C**holangitis	
M **M**ucocele		

Charcot's triad for cholangitis

3 Cs

C **C**olour change (jaundice)
C **C**olicky RUQ pain
C **C**hills and fever

Gastrectomy

Complications

3 Ds

D **D**umping syndrome
D **D**iarrhoea
D **D**eficiency of vitamin B_{12}

Diverticular disease

Causes and risk factors

RAC

R **R**efined low-fibre diet
A ↑ **A**ge
C **C**onnective tissue disorders

Complications of diverticulosis

POUCH

P **P**ainful diverticulitis/**P**erforation
O **O**bstruction of colon
U **PU**s formation – peri-colic abscess
C **C**onnections formed, ie fistulae in colon–small bowel or colon–vagina or colon–bladder (pneumaturia ± intractable UTIs)
H **H**aemorrhage (caused by vessel erosion)

Intestinal obstruction

Symptoms

Preventing **V**accinations **C**auses **D**isease

P **P**ain – severe and gripping colicky pain with periods of ease, located in the central (small intestine) or lower abdomen (large intestine)
V **V**omiting
C **C**onstipation – absolute, ie failure to pass either stool or flatus
D **D**istension – occurs more in large intestine obstruction

Breast disease

Risk factors

BREAST

B **B**RCA genes/**B**abyless, ie nulliparity/**B**reast-feeding avoided
R **R**eplacement therapy with hormones (HRT)
E **E**arly menarche/**E**xposure to oestrogen for long period
A **A**ge ↑
S **S**ize is large, ie obesity
T **T**rend in family (important in 5–10% cases)

Differential diagnosis of a breast lump

FBC

F **F**ibroadenoma
B **B**reast cyst
C **C**arcinoma of breast

Investigation of a breast lump

The buzzword here is **TRIPLE ASSESSMENT**, which consists of:

HRT

H **H**istory and Examination
R **R**adiology: ultrasound or mammography
T **T**issue diagnosis: cytology or biopsy

Remembering from Chapter 10 that HRT increases the risk of developing breast cancer.

Lumps and bumps

Examining

3 **S**s, 3 **C**s, 3**T**s and the **F**'er

3Ss **S**ite, **S**ize, **S**hape
3Cs **C**olour, **C**onsistency, **C**ontour
3Ts **T**enderness, **T**ethering, **T**ransillumination
F'er **F**luctuance

Hernias

Groin lump: differential diagnosis

Surgeons **L**ike **T**o **M**anage **V**arious **H**ernias

S **S**permatic cord (lipoma, hydrocoele)/**S**kin (sebaceous cyst)
L **L**ymph nodes
T **T**esticle (ectopic, undescended)
M **M**uscle (psoas abscess)
V **V**ascular (femoral artery aneurysm, saphena varyx)
H **H**ernias (inguinal, femoral)

Inguinal hernia: causes and risk factors

Congenital: Abdominal contents enter the inguinal canal through a patent processus vaginalis
Acquired: ↑ intra-abdominal pressure together with muscle and transversalis fascia weakness; causes for this can be recalled by **CANALS**:

C **C**hronic cough, eg COPD, asthma/**C**onstipation
A **A**scites
N I**N**creased muscular effort
A **A**ge ↑
L **L**arge size – obesity
S **S**ex: males more common/**S**training due to bladder outflow obstruction (prostatic disease)

Femoral hernia: epidemiology

FEMoral hernias occur more commonly in **FEM**ales (female:male is 4:1)

Abdominal wall hernias

APIL (sounds like an apple!)

A **A**nterior hernias: epigastric, incisional, Spigelian, supravesical, umbilical
P **P**elvic hernias: obturator, perineal, sciatic
I **I**nguinal hernias: indirect, direct, femoral
L **L**umbar hernias: inferior lumbar triangle (Petit), superior lumbar triangle

Incisional hernia: causes and risk factors

INCISE

I   **I**ncreasing age
N   **N**utrition inadequate – protein and vitamin/mineral deficiencies
C   **C**ytotoxic drugs/**C**orticosteroids
I   **I**ncision type, eg midline
S   **S**uture material/**S**urgical skill
E   **E**xposure to radiation – radiotherapy

Scrotal swelling

Questions that need answering (when examining patient)

TEST

T   Is it **T**ender?
E   Can you **E**xceed the lump ie get above it?
S   Is the lump **S**eparate from the testis ie can you identify the testis and epididymis?
T   Does it **T**ransilluminate?

Differential diagnosis

TWO TESTES

T   **T**rauma
W **W**aricocele (actually begins with V!)
O   **O**rchitis
T   **T**umour of testis
E   **E**pididymitis
S   **S**permatocele
T   **T**orsion of testis
E   **HE**rnia – indirect inguinal
S   **S**erous fluid collection within tunica vaginalis, ie hydrocele

Unilateral leg swelling

Causes

in**CL. VAT**

C **C**ellulitis
L **L**ymphoedema
V **V**enous – varicose veins, venous thrombosis, obstruction to venous return
A **A**llergy
T **T**rauma – ruptured Baker's cyst

DVT

The mechanisms that lead to venous thrombosis are summed up with **Virchow's triad**. To appreciate this, one must remember that a DVT is a formation of a thrombus within the deep veins (most commonly of the calf or thigh) and these constitute a part of the **VaSC**ular system.

Virchow's triad

V **V**essel wall injury
S **S**tasis, ie blood flow disturbance
C **C**omposition of blood changes, ie hypercoagulability

Causes and risk factors

POPADOMS

P **P**ost-surgery (especially pelvic and orthopaedic)
O **O**CP use
P **P**regnancy/**P**olycythaemia
A **A**ctive malignancy/**A**ir travel (long haul flight)
D **D**ehydration/**D**eficiency of protein C or antithrombin III; thrombophilia disorders
O **O**besity
M **M**ovement restricted for long periods, ie immobility
S **S**moking

Limb ischaemia

Symptoms and Signs of acute limb ischaemia

6 Ps

P **P**ale
P **P**ulseless
P **P**araesthesia
P **P**ainful
P **P**aralysis
P 'Perishingly' cold

Varicose veins

Signs and symptom

AEIOUS

A **A**ching legs
E **E**czema
I **I**tching/**I**nfection
O **O**edema
U **U**lcers
S **S**ight: 'my legs are ugly'

Leg ulcers

Causes (majority are venous)

ISCHAEMIA

I **I**schaemia
S **S**yphilis
C **C**onnective tissue disorders, eg RA
H **H**aematological disorders e.g. sickle cell disease
A **A**buse
E **E**ndocrine, eg DM
M **M**alignancy, eg squamous cell carcinoma, basal cell carcinoma
I **I**nfected injury
A **A**-V fistula

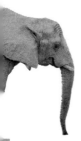

18. Trauma and orthopaedics

Anatomy

Upper limb

Rotator cuff muscles

SITS

S **S**upraspinatus (abductor)
I **I**nfraspinatus (external rotator)
T **T**eres minor (external rotator)
S **S**ubscapularis (internal rotator)

Serratus anterior innervation

SALT

Serratus **A**nterior = **L**ong **T**horacic nerve

Latissimus dorsi

Lady **D**iedre between **T**wo **MAJORS**

An old favourite! This reminds us that the **L**atissumus **D**orsi muscle is attached on the humerus; on the floor of the bicipital groove with the tendon between the attachments of the pectoralis **major** and teres **major**.

Brachial plexus subunits

Richard **T**urner **D**rinks **C**old **B**everages

R **R**oots
T **T**runks
D **D**ivisions
C **C**ords
B **B**ranches

Numbers of each of the subunits

5-3-2-3-5

5 Roots
3 Trunks
2 Divisions
3 Cords
5 Branches

It is the same backwards and forwards!

Cubital fossa contents

Please **R**emember **B**e **B**rave **M**edically

From lateral to medial:

P **P**osterior interosseus nerve
R **R**adial nerve
B **B**iceps tendon
B **B**rachial artery
M **M**edian nerve

Elbow: muscles that flex it

The **3 Bs B**end the el**B**ow

B **B**rachialis
B **B**iceps
B **B**rachioradialis

Arm fracture

Nerves affected by humerus fracture location

ARM fracture

From superior to inferior:

A **A**xillary: head of humerus
R **R**adial: mid-shaft
M **M**edian: supracondylar

Interossei muscles of the hand: actions of the dorsal versus palmar muscles

There are 4 palmar and 4 dorsal interossei and all are innervated by the ulnar nerve.

Remember **Pad** and **Dab**:

The **P**almar **ad**duct and the **D**orsal **ab**duct (use your hand to **dab** with a **pad**)

The carpal bones

The eight small bones of the wrist are arranged in two rows of four. By following the proposed format, a logical method of remembering them can be seen: in the proximal row, follow the bones from **lateral** to **medial**:

Some **L**ecturers **T**each **P**roperly, **H**owever **C**ountless **T**each **T**erribly

S **S**caphoid
L **L**unate
T **T**riquetrium
P **P**isiform

Then the distal row, follow the opposite format, ie from **medial** to **lateral**:

H **H**amate
C **C**apitate
T **T**rapezoid
T **T**rapezium

Osteoblast versus osteoclast

Osteo**B**last **B**uilds bone

Osteo**C**last **C**onsumes bone

Musculocutaneous nerve

Muscles supplied

BBC

B   **B**iceps brachii
B   **B**rachialis
C   **C**oracobrachialis

Radial nerve

Muscles supplied

The radial nerve supplies all the **BEST** muscles

B   **B**rachioradialis
E   **E**xtensors
S   **S**upinator
T   **T**riceps

Ulnar nerve

Muscles supplied

MAFFIA

M   **M**edial two lumbricals
A   **A**dductor pollicis
F   **F**lexor carpi ulnaris
F   **F**lexor digitorum profundus
I   **I**nterossei
A   **A**bductor digiti minimi and hypothenar eminence

Relationship of nerves to arteries in the upper limb

When remembering the relationship of the peripheral nerves to their arteries, think that the ulnar nerve is 'ulnar' to the ulnar artery and the radial nerve is 'radial' to the radial artery.

Hand nerve lesions

DR CUMAR

Wrist **D**rop = **R**adial nerve

Claw hand = **U**lnar nerve

Median nerve = **A**pe hand (or **R**eligious person's hand, ie preacher)

Supination versus pronation

SOUP and POUR

SOUPination: supination is to turn your arm palm up, as if holding a bowl of **soup**

POURnation: pronation is to turn your arm with the palm down, as if **pour**ing soup out of bowl

Lower limb

Safest quadrant on buttock to insert injection

Shut **UP** and **BUTT OUT**

The **UP**per **OUT**er quadrant of the **BUTT**ock is the safest place to inject as it avoids hitting the sciatic nerve

Hip and thigh

Lateral rotators

Please **G**o **O**ut, **G**us **O**perates **Q**uietly

P   **P**iriformis
G   **G**emellus superior
O   **O**bturator internus
G   **G**emellus inferior
O   **O**bturator externus
Q   **Q**uadratus femoris

Adductor muscles of thigh

Post-**G**raduates **L**ove their **B**achelor **O**f **M**edicine

P **P**ectineus
G **G**racilis
L Adductor **L**ongus
B Adductor **B**revis
O **O**bturator nerve innervates all these muscles expect for the pectineus (femoral nerve). Part of the adductor magnus is supplied by the sciatic nerve
M Adductor **M**agnus

As well as adducting, these muscles are important in fixing the hip joint and for normal gait

Posterior compartment of thigh

By **T**onight **M**emorise **M**ap

B **B**iceps femoris
T Semi**T**endinosus
M Semi**M**embranosus
M Adductor **M**agnus (hamstring portion)

Innervation of thigh relevant to compartment

MAP OF Scilly

Medial compartment: **O**bturator nerve

Anterior compartment: **F**emoral nerve

Posterior compartment: **Sci**atic nerve

Perineal versus peroneal

Per**IN**eal is **IN** between the legs

Per**ON**eal is **ON** the leg

Lower leg bones

Getting confused between your tibia and fibula? The **TIB**ia is the **T**hick **I**nner **B**one whilst the **F**ibu**L**a is the **F**iner, **L**ateral bone

Tarsal tunnel contents

Too **D**issect **A**ppropriately **N**eed **H**elp

From superior to inferior:

T **T**ibialis posterior
D Flexor **D**igitorum longus
A Posterior tibial **A**rtery
N Tibial **N**erve
H Flexor **H**allucis longus

Medial malleolus: order of tendons, artery and nerve behind it

Tom, **D**ick **A**nd **N**ot **H**arry

From anterior to posterior:

T **T**ibialis posterior
D Flexor **D**igitorum longus
A Tibial **A**rtery
N Posterior tibial **N**erve
H Flexor **H**allucis longus

Clinical conditions

Painful neck

Differentials

Jock **STRAP**

J **J**erking back of the head and neck, ie whiplash
S **S**pondylosis/**S**pondylolisthesis of cervical discs
T **T**orticollis (spasmodic/infantile)
R Cervical **R**ib
A **A**bnormal posture
P **P**rolapsed cervical disc

Painful arc syndrome

This is pain on abduction between 45° and 160°

Causes

ARC

A **A**cromioclavicular (AC) joint osteoarthritis
R **R**otator cuff muscle tendinitis, ie supraspinatus tendinitis
C **C**alcifying tendinitis

Carpal tunnel syndrome

Causes and risk factors

CARPAL

C **C**ardiac failure/**C**ombined OCP use
A **A**cromegaly
R **R**enal disorder – nephrotic syndrome/**R**aised glucose levels; DM
P **P**regnancy/**P**oor thyroid function; hypo-thyroidism
A **A**rthritis of the wrist (rheumatoid, osteoarthritis)
L **L**arge size – obesity

Special tests to detect carpal tunnel syndrome

TINel's sign

TINgling sensation after **T**apping on **T**raumatised nerve in carpal **T**unnel syndrome

Phalen's test

Maximal **Ph**lexion (flexion) of the wrist for 1 min may cause symptoms.

Motor assessment

Test the power of the muscles that are innervated by the median nerve

LOAF

L **L**ateral two lumbricals – difficult to test

O **O**pponens pollicis – oppose the patient's thumb and the little finger and ask them to stop you pulling the fingers apart

A **A**bductor pollicis brevis – place dorsum of hand on a flat surface and ask the patient to lift their thumb to the ceiling against resistance

F **F**lexor pollicis brevis – not an independent muscle (innervation varies)

To remember that these are the **Me**dian nerve muscles, think '**Me**at **LOAF**'

Lordosis versus kyphosis versus scoliosis

Lordosis: **L**umbar curvature increased, **L**ower down on spine

KYphosis: **HY** up on the spine causing anterior curvature/**K**lose to caput

Scoliosis: **S**-shaped spine causing lateral curvature

Painful back

Differentials

TOMS DIScman

T **T**umours of spine

O **O**steoporosis/**O**steomalacia

M **M**echanical

S **S**pondylolisthesis

D **D**isc prolapse/lesion

I **I**nfection

S **S**tenosis of lumbar spine/lateral recess (due to facet joint osteoarthritis)

Differential diagnosis of a limp

STARTSS HOT

S **S**eptic joint
T **T**umour
A **A**vascular necrosis (Legg–Calve–Perthe's)
R **R**heumatoid arthritis/juvenile rheumatoid arthritis
T **T**uberculosis
S **S**ickle cell disease
S **S**lipped upper femoral epiphysis (SUFE)

H **H**SP
O **O**steomyelitis
T **T**rauma

Painful knee

Differentials

ABCDE

A **A**rthritis – rheumatoid and osteoarthritis
B **B**ipartite patella
C **C**hondromalacia patellae
D **D**eformity of patella, ie recurrent subluxation of patella
E **E**xcessive lateral pressure syndrome

Swollen knee

Differentials

TOMBOLA

T **T**orn or injured (cruciates/collaterals) ligaments
O **O**steoarthritis
M **M**eniscal cysts
B **B**ursitis – prepatellar bursitis ('housemaid's knee') most common
O **O**steochondritis dissecans
L **L**oose bodies in the knee
A **A**bnormal patella, ie dislocated patella

Genu valgum versus genu varum

Genu val**GUM** (knock-knee): knees are **GUM**med together

Genu **Var**um (bowleg) is when the knees are far apart as **Far** rhymes with **Var** so knees are **far** apart

Pes cavus versus pes planus

Pes **C**avus: **C**law foot

Pes **PL**anus: **L**ow arched foot, ie flat foot

Hammer toes

Hamm**E**r

H   **H**yperflexed at PIP joint
E   **E**xtended at DIP joint
E   **E**xtended at MTP joint

Hallux valgus

Hallux va**L**gus

L   **L**ateral deviation of toe at MTP joint

Painful heel

Differentials

DRs **PACT**

D   **D**iseases of the calcaneum
R   **R**upture of calcaneal tendon
P   **P**lantar fasciitis/**P**ost-calcaneal bursitis
A   **A**rthritis of subtalar joint
C   **C**alcaneal paratendinitis
T   **T**ender heel pad

Osteomyelitis

Causes and risk factors

I PAID

I Infection (bacterial)
P Prostheses
A Anaemia – sickle-cell
I Immunosuppression
D Drugs – IV use

Complications

FIBRE

F Fractures
I Intraosseous (Brodie) abscesses
B Bacteraemia
R Reactive amyloidosis
E Endocarditis

Osteosarcoma

Risk factors and features

Osteosarcoma is the most common **PRIM**ary malignant **TUM**our of bones

PRIM TUM

P Paget's disease
R Radiation
I Infection of the bone
M Males (more common in)
T Ten-Twenty five years of age most commonly affected
U Uncommon – incidence = three/million
M Mutations of oncogenes – retinoblastoma, Li–Fraumeni syndrome

Charcot's joints

Causes

Diabetic People Lose Sensation, Can Traumatise

Peripheral:

- **D** **D**iabetic neuropathy
- **P** **P**eripheral nerve injuries
- **L** **L**eprosy

Central:

- **S** **S**yringomyelia/**S**pina bifida
- **C** **C**auda equina syndrome, eg secondary to myelomeningocele
- **T** **T**abes dorsalis

Management of chronic orthopaedic conditions: general rule of thumb

3Ps

- **P** **P**ain relief
- **P** **P**hysiotherapy
- **P** **P**erform surgery

Trauma

Soft tissue injuries

Treatment

RICE (protocol employed in the 1st 24 hours following the injury)

- **R** **R**est
- **I** **I**ce
- **C** **C**ompression
- **E** **E**levation

Compartment syndrome

Signs and symptoms

All Ps

P   **P**ain out of **P**roportion to injury
P   **P**ain on **P**assive flexion
P   **P**alpate tense compartment
P   **P**allor, **P**aralysis, **P**ulseless, **P**araesthesia (all these are seen in the late stage of the condition)

Fractures

Fracture types

Star wars fans can easily recall the various types of fractures

Go C3PO

G   **G**reenstick
O   **O**pen
C   **C**omplete
C   **C**losed
C   **C**omminuted
P   **P**artial
O   **O**ther

Management

Depends on: type of fracture, nature of injury, age and medical condition of patient.

In general, the **6 Rs** should be followed:

R   **R**esuscitate – ATLS Management: **A**irways, **B**reathing, **C**irculation, **D**isability, **E**xposure
R   **R**adiology – X-rays: AP and lateral/joint above and below
R   **R**educe
R   **R**estrict, ie fixate
R   **R**emain patient, ie wait
R   **R**ehabilitate

Glasgow Coma Scale (GCS)

This is used to assess the level of consciousness and it consists of three parts. The minimum score is 3 and the maximum is 15

E$_4$ **V**$_5$ **M**$_6$

E **E**yes opening (1–4) ('eyes' has 4 letters)
V **V**erbal response (1–5) ('V' represents 5 in Roman numerals)
M **M**otor response (1–6) (M6 is a famous motorway in the UK)

Numbers indicate the minimum and maximum degrees of deficit within each category. Remember if the GCS is less than **eight**, intub**ate**.

AVPU score

Level of consciousness can be more rapidly assessed by **AVPU** score:

A **A**lert?
V Responds to **V**oice?
P Responds to **P**ain?
U **U**nresponsive?

In addition, remember to check if **PERL** is seen:

Pupils **E**qual and **R**eactive to **L**ight

Index

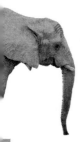

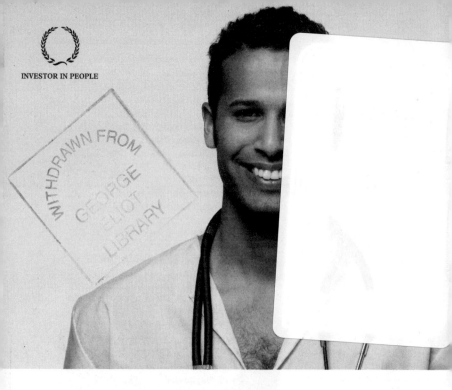
Independent Financial Advice for **Doctors**
from like-minded professionals

If you're hard working and successful in a demanding career, you want to be sure that your financial affairs are just as well organised. What's often missing is a source of reliable advice: an independent contact with more know-how than the usual banker or insurance salesman. MLP is one of the foremost independent financial advisers in Europe. Our clients are, almost invariably, professionals. Our focus on professional groups has enabled us to develop financial planning concepts for

- **Investments**
- **Retirement**
- **Property ownership**
- **Protection** that can be tailor-made to individual aspirations

To achieve these objectives, MLP financial consultants themselves come from an academic background. They are also required to complete intensive and on-going training.
So, rather than settle for second best, look for quality advice.

To arrange a free consultation with MLP contact us at **info@mlpuk.co.uk** or call **0845 30 10 999**

HEAD OFFICE 12 Bedford Square
London WC1B 3JA
*MLP has offices in London,
Birmingham, Edinburgh and Bristol*

MLP Private Finance PLC is authorised and
regulated by the Financial Services Authority

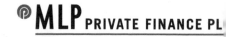

MLP PRIVATE FINANCE PL

www.mlp-plc.co.uk